NMR and Chemistry

An introduction to the
Fourier transform–multinuclear era

NMR and Chemistry
An introduction to the
Fourier transform–multinuclear era

J. W. Akitt

School of Chemistry
University of Leeds

Second Edition

London   New York
CHAPMAN AND HALL

First published 1973 by
Chapman and Hall Ltd
11 New Fetter Lane, London EC4P 4EE

Published in the USA by
Chapman and Hall
733 Third Avenue, New York NY 10017

Second edition 1983

© 1983 J. W. Akitt

Printed in Great Britain by
J. W. Arrowsmith Ltd, Bristol

ISBN 0 412 24010 6 (cased)
ISBN 0 412 24020 3 (Science Paperback)

British Library Cataloguing in Publication Data	Library of Congress Cataloging in Publication Data

Akitt, J. W.
    NMR and chemistry. – 2nd ed.
    1. Nuclear magnetic resonance spectroscopy
    I. Title
538'.362   QC762
ISBN 0–412–24010–6
ISBN 0–412–24020–3 Pbk
	Akitt, J. W.
	    NMR and chemistry.
	    Bibliography: p.
	    Includes index.
	    1. Nuclear magnetic resonance spectroscopy.
	I. Title. II. Title: N.M.R. and chemistry.
	QD96.N8A37 1983 538'.362 83–1773
	ISBN 0–412–24010–6
	ISBN 0–412–24020–3 (pbk.)

Contents

Preface to the First Edition

About 20 years have elapsed since chemists started to take an interest in nuclear magnetic resonance spectroscopy. In the intervening period it has proved to be a very powerful and informative branch of spectroscopy, so much so that today most research groups have access to one or more spectrometers and the practising chemist can expect constantly to encounter references to the technique. There is a considerable number of textbooks available on the subject but these are invariably written primarily either for the specialist or for the graduate student who is starting to use the technique in his research. The author has, however, always felt that a place existed for a non-specialist text written for the undergraduate student giving an introduction to the subject which embraced the whole NMR scene and which would serve as a basis for later specialisation in any of the three main branches of chemistry.

With this in mind the book has been written in two sections. The first covers the theory using a straightforward non-mathematical approach which nevertheless introduces some of the most modern descriptions of the various phenomena. The text is illustrated by specific examples where necessary. The second section is devoted to showing how the technique is used and gives some more complex examples illustrating for instance its use for structure determination and for measurements of reaction rates and mechanisms. A few problems have been included but the main purpose of the book is to demonstrate the many and varied present uses of NMR rather than to teach the student how to analyse a spectrum in detail. This is done best if it is done concurrently with a student's own research.

I am indebted to Dr K. D. Crosbie, Professor N. N. Greenwood, Dr B. E. Mann, and to Professor D. H. Whiffen who read and criticised the manuscript and to many former colleagues at Newcastle-upon-Tyne for encouragement and for some of the examples used in the text. I also give grateful acknowledgement to Varian Associates Ltd. for permission to reproduced the spectra in Figs 15, 17, 26, 27, 66 and 75 and to Bruker-Spectrospin Ltd. for permission to reproduce the spectra in Figs 49, 50, 63, 64 and 75.

Leeds,   **J.W.A.**
January, 1972

Preface to the Second Edition

It is just ten years since I wrote the preface to the first edition of this book. The intervening decade has, however, seen such an explosive development of the subject that it has changed almost out of all recognition. Certainly some material has had to be completely replaced by new and the text has had to be extensively rewritten to accommodate current concepts. The first edition contained a mention of Fourier transform techniques, and of superconducting magnets, and these two fields have both developed extremely rapidly because it was realized that they would make possible some real advances in chemical research. The new ^{13}C spectroscopy of organic molecules on the one hand increased the scope of the technique for structural determination, and high field proton spectroscopy on the other enabled the problem of the solution structure of large, biologically important molecules to be tackled. It was also increasingly realized that the Fourier transform pulse techniques allowed precise manipulation of nuclear spins so that many different new relaxation or double resonance experiments became possible. Such advances have also proved to be informative when applied to the less popular nuclei and so multinuclear flexibility was introduced into the new, powerful NMR spectrometers, which can, in principle, carry out most likely experiments with every magnetically active nucleus in the periodic table.

Development has, however, not stopped here. The difficult field of the high resolution study of solid samples is being successfully ploughed; the separation of shift and coupling parameters in a two-dimensional experiment is now possible and the biologists have started to look at somewhat unusual samples such as anaesthetized live rats.

One particularly interesting development which is being vigorously

pursued is that of whole body imaging. It has proved possible to map
out the proton density of the water in the body using pulsed NMR
techniques in conjunction with specially contoured magnetic fields.
This gives a thin cross-section of selected parts of human subjects which
can be obtained quickly and safely and gives information which is likely
to be complementary to that obtained by X-rays. Thus our technique
has expanded and moved into an area which can be seen to be vital to
the whole of mankind. Practising spectroscopists will of course be able
to point to many areas where NMR has proved invaluable to science
and industry, and so to mankind in general. Such advances are unfortunately not immediately obvious to the public at large, and we
should welcome the advent of whole body imaging, as a visible testament
to the utility of pure science. The physicists who first detected nuclear
magnetic resonances are unlikely to have had concern for anything but
the details their investigations revealed about the nucleus of the atom.
When it became apparent to chemists that the technique was capable of
giving uniquely valuable information about the structure of molecules,
then their demands led to the development of a spectrometer industry
serving academic and industrial science: their quest for higher sensitivity
led to the Fourier transform technique and this now is set to lead us
into a new medical based industry. Such developments should be well
pondered by those who would constrain pure scientific research.

   I have left the general plan of the book much as in the first edition;
theory, followed by examples of the use of the technique which serve
also to reinforce the theory. The technique is approached as primarily a
pulse spectrometry but it has proved necessary to retain mention of the
old continuous wave methods. Continuous wave equipment is still with
us and even the most advanced pulse spectrometer makes use of a
continuous wave technique to adjust the magnetic field homogeneity
and to provide a field-frequency lock.

   I am again indebted to many colleagues for assistance and comments;
Dr R. J. Bushby for Fig. 9.17, Professor N. N. Greenwood, Dr O. W.
Howarth of Warwick University for Fig. 9.22, Dr J. D. Kennedy for
Figs 9.37–9.39 and 9.53, Dr B. E. Mann of Sheffield University for
Fig. 9.32, Professeur G. J. Martin of the Université de Nantes for
supplying the spectra to illustrate Fig. 4.20, Dr A. Römer of Cologne
University for Figs 9.14–9.16 and Professor B. L. Shaw for Figs 9.25,
9.44–9.46. I am doubly indebted to Dr Kennedy for reading the entire
manuscript and for suggesting some valuable additions. I also give
grateful acknowledgement to Varian International AG for permission
to reproduce the spectra in Figs 3.3, 3.5, 3.14, 3.17, 9.2–9.10, 9.13;

to Bruker-Spectrospin Ltd for permission to reproduce diagrams and spectra in their application notes as Figs 7.4, 7.5, 8.9–8.16; to Heyden and Son Ltd (John Wiley and Sons, Inc.) for permission to reproduce Figs 4.4, 4.17, 4.20, 8.4, 8.5 and Table 7.1; to the American Chemical Society for permission to reproduce Figs 3.22, 4.19, 7.6, 8.3, 9.20, 9.21, 9.27, 9.28, 9.34, 9.35, 9.42, 9.43, 9.48 and 9.50; to Academic Press for permission to reproduce Figs 5.9, 5.10, 7.10, 7.15, 7.16, 7.17 and 9.41; to the American Association for the Advancement of Science for permission to reproduce Figs 8.6 and 8.7; to the Royal Society of Chemistry for permission to reproduce Figs 3.11, 7.2, 8.2, 8.8 and 9.23; to the American Institute of Physics for permission to reproduce Figs 6.2, 8.17, 9.29, 9.30, 9.31, 9.36 and 9.51; to Elsevier Sequoia SA for permission to reproduce Fig. 9.26; and the Royal Society for permission to reproduce Fig. 3.21.

Leeds   **J.W.A.**
March 1982

1
The Theory of Nuclear Magnetization

1.1   The properties of the nucleus of an atom

The chemist normally thinks of the atomic nucleus as possessing only
mass and charge and is concerned more with the interactions of the
electrons which surround the nucleus, neutralize its charge and give
rise to the chemical properties of the atom. Nuclei however possess
several other properties which are of importance to chemistry and to
understand how we use them it is necessary to know something more
about them.

Nuclei of certain isotopes possess intrinsic angular momentum or
spin, of total magnitude $\hbar[I(I+1)]^{1/2}$. The largest measurable
component of this angular moment is $I\hbar$, where I is the nuclear spin
quantum number and $\hbar$ is the reduced Plancks' constant, $h/2\pi$. I may
have integral or half integral values $(0, 1/2, 1, 3/2 \ldots)$, the actual value
depending upon the isotope. If $I = 0$ the nucleus has no angular
momentum. Since I is quantized, several discrete values of angular
momentum may be observable and their magnitudes are given by $\hbar m$,
where the quantum number m can take the values $I, I-1, I-2 \ldots -I$.
There are thus $2I + 1$ equally spaced spin states of a nucleus with
angular momentum quantum number I.

A nucleus with spin also has an associated magnetic moment μ. We
can naively consider this as arising from the effect of the spinning
nuclear charge which at its periphery forms a current loop. We define
the components of μ associated with the different spin states as $m\mu/I$,
so that μ also has $2I + 1$ components. In the absence of an external
magnetic field the spin states all possess the same potential energy, but
take different values if a field is applied. The origin of the NMR

technique lies in these energy differences, though we must defer further discussion of this until we have defined some other basic nuclear properties.

The magnetic moment and angular momentum behave as if they were parallel or antiparallel vectors. It is convenient to define a ratio between them which is called the magnetogyric ratio, γ.

$$\gamma = \frac{2\pi}{h} \frac{\mu}{I} = \frac{\mu}{I\hbar} \tag{1.1}$$

γ has a characteristic value for each magnetically active nucleus and is positive for parallel and negative for antiparallel vectors.

If $I > 1/2$ the nucleus possesses in addition an electric quadrupole moment, Q. This means that the distribution of charge in the nucleus is non-spherical and that it can interact with electric field gradients arising from the electric charge distribution in the molecule. This interaction provides a means by which the nucleus can exchange energy with the molecule in which it is situated and affects certain NMR spectra profoundly.

Some nuclei have $I = 0$. Important examples are the major isotopes ^{12}C and ^{16}O which are both magnetically inactive — a fact which leads to considerable simplification of the spectra of organic molecules. It is instructive to consider the meaning of zero spin. Such nuclei are free to rotate in the classical sense and so form a current loop but have no associated magnetic moment. We must not confuse the idea of quantum mechanical 'spin' with classical rotation however. The nucleons, that is the particles such as neutrons and protons which make up the nucleus, possess intrinsic spin in the same way as do electrons in atoms. Nucleons of opposite spin can pair, just as do electrons, though they can only pair with nucleons of the same kind. Thus in a nucleus with even numbers of both protons and neutrons all the spins are paired and $I = 0$. If there are odd numbers of either or of both, then the spin is non-zero, though its actual value depends upon orbital type internucleon interactions. Thus we build up a picture of the nucleus in which the different resolved angular momenta in a magnetic field imply different nucleon arrangements within the nucleus, the number of spin states depending upon the number of possible arrangements. If we add to this picture the concept that s bonding electrons have finite charge density within the nucleus and become partly nucleon in character, then we can see that these spin states might be perturbed by the hybridization of the bonding electrons and that information derived from the nuclear states might lead indirectly to information about the electronic system and its chemistry.

The properties of the most important magnetic isotopes of each element are summarized in Fig. 1.1, which is set out as a periodic table. Each panel of the table contains the spectrometer frequency for a 23.48 kilogauss magnet (2.348 tesla −this field is chosen since it gives a frequency of 100 MHz for ^{1}H), the isotope number of a main active isotope, the spin quantum number I, the nuclear quadrupole moment Q where $I > 1/2$, the natural abundance rounded off to two significant figures, and the receptivity, which is a relative sensitivity figure used to compare signal areas theoretically obtainable at a given magnetic field strength for different nuclei and taking into account both the different magnetic moments and the different natural abundances. Two receptivity figures may be encountered, D^P, the one used here taking ^{1}H as unity, or one relative to ^{13}C for the less receptive nuclei and called D^c. The resonance line heights of nuclei giving resonances of the same width will be in the ratio of these receptivity figures. If more than one isotope of an element has found use in NMR then this is shown by an ‡, except in the case of deuterium, ^{2}H, sometimes written, D, which is important enough to warrant a separate panel of its own.

The usefulness of a nucleus depends in the first place upon the chemical importance of the atom it characterizes and then upon its receptivity. Thus the extreme importance of carbon spectroscopy for understanding the structures of organic molecules has led to technical developments which have overcome the disadvantages of the low receptivity of its magnetically active nucleus, ^{13}C. However, up to quite recently the problems associated with low receptivity had meant that most effort had been expended on relatively few nuclei of high receptivity of which the proton is the most important (proton $\equiv$ ^{1}H − the term proton is commonly used by NMR spectroscopists when discussing the nucleus of neutral hydrogen) since it is a constituent of the majority of organic and many inorganic compounds and gives access to the physical study of diverse systems. Many studies have also been made with boron ^{11}B, for instance in the boron hydrides and carboranes, with fluorine ^{19}F in the vast array of fluoro organics and inorganics and with phosphorus ^{31}P in its many inorganic and biochemical guises. Today, however, the developments which have led to the much more difficult ^{13}C spectroscopy being commonplace mean that virtually the whole of the periodic table is open to study by NMR spectroscopy and many examples will be given in later chapters.

	^7Li	^9Be		^1H	^2H	^3He
Frequency MHz	38.8	14.0		100.0	15.3	76.2
Spin I	3/2	3/2		1/2	1	1/2
Q	−0.03	0.052		—	0.0027	—
Abundance %	93*‡	100		100	0.015	10^{-4}
receptivity D^p	0.27	1.4×10^{-2}		1	1.5×10^{-6}	5.8×10^{-7}

	^{23}Na	^{25}Mg
Frequency MHz	26.5	6.1
Spin I	3/2	5/2
Q	0.15	0.22
Abundance %	100	10
receptivity D^p	9.3×10^{-2}	2.7×10^{-4}

	^{39}K	^{43}Ca	^{45}Sc	^{47}Ti	^{51}V	^{53}Cr	^{55}Mn	^{57}Fe
Frequency MHz	4.7	6.7	24.3	5.6	26.3	5.6	24.7	3.2
Spin I	3/2	7/2	7/2	5/2	7/2	3/2	5/2	1/2
Q	0.11	0.2	−0.22	0.29	0.04	−0.03	0.55	—
Abundance %	93	0.13	100	7.8	100	9.54	100	2.2
receptivity D^p	4.7×10^{-4}	9.3×10^{-6}	0.301	1.5×10^{-4}	0.381	8.6×10^{-5}	0.175	7.4×10^{-7}

	^{87}Rb	^{87}Sr	^{89}Y	^{91}Zr	^{93}Nb	^{95}Mo	Tc	^{101}Ru
Frequency MHz	32.7	4.3	4.9	9.3	24.4	6.5		4.9
Spin I	3/2	9/2	1/2	5/2	9/2	5/2		5/2
Q	0.13	0.2	—	?	−0.2	0.12		?
Abundance %	27	7	100	11	100	16		17
receptivity D^p	4.9×10^{-2}	1.9×10^{-4}	1.2×10^{-4}	1×10^{-3}	0.482	5.1×10^{-4}		1.7×10^{-4}

	^{133}Cs	^{137}Ba	^{139}La	^{177}Hf	^{181}Ta	^{183}W	^{187}Re	^{189}Os
Frequency MHz	13.1	11.1	14.1	3.0	12.0	4.1	22.8	7.8
Spin I	7/2	3/2	7/2	7/2	7/2	1/2	5/2	3/2
Q	−0.003	0.2	0.21	3	3	—	2.6	0.8
Abundance %	100	11	100	18	100	14	63	16
receptivity D^p	4.7×10^{-2}	8.0×10^{-4}	5.9×10^{-2}	1.2×10^{-4}	3.6×10^{-2}	1.0×10^{-5}	8.6×10^{-2}	3.8×10^{-4}

	Ce	^{141}Pr	^{143}Nd	Pm	^{147}Sm
Frequency MHz		27.0	6.3		3.5
Spin I		5/2	7/2		7/2
Q		−0.059	−0.48		−0.208
Abundance %		100	12		15
receptivity D^p		0.26	3.2×10^{-4}		1.3×10^{-4}

*Of variable abundance either normally or due to commerical separation

Figure 1.1   Table of main naturally occurring magnetically active isotopes. The table shows only one nucleus for each element, but it should be borne in mind that many elements have several magnetically active isotopes. (‡) Some of importance are ^6Li, ^{10}B, ^{15}N, ^{37}Cl, ^{79}Br, ^{115}Sn, ^{131}Xe, ^{201}Hg and ^{204}Tl. The NMR frequency in a magnetic field of 23.48 kG (2.348T) is given to the nearest 0.1 MHz. This figure is proportional to the magnetogyric ratio γ. Spin quantum number I,

1.2   The nucleus in a magnetic field

If we place a nucleus in a magnetic field $\mathbf{B}_0$ it can take up $2I + 1$ orientations in the field, each one at a particular angle θ to the field direction and associated with a different potential energy. The energy of a nucleus of magnetic moment μ in field $\mathbf{B}_0$ is $-\mu_z \mathbf{B}_0$, where μ_z is the component of μ in the field direction. The energy of the various

	^{11}B	^{13}C	^{14}N	^{17}O	^{19}F	^{21}Ne
	32.1	25.1	7.2	13.6	94.1	7.8
	3/2	1/2	1	5/2	1/2	3/2
	0.036	–	0.016	−0.026	–	?
	80*‡	1.1*	99.6‡	0.037*‡	100	0.26
	0.133	1.8×10^{-4}	1.0×10^{-3}	1.1×10^{-5}	0.83	6.3×10^{-6}

	^{27}Al	^{29}Si	^{31}P	^{33}S	^{35}Cl	Ar
	26.1	19.9	40.5	7.7	9.8	
	5/2	1/2	1/2	3/2	3/2	
	0.149	–	–	−0.064	−0.079	
	100	4.7*	100	0.76*	75.5‡	
	0.21	3.7×10^{-4}	6.6×10^{-2}	1.7×10^{-5}	3.6×10^{-3}	

^{59}Co	^{61}Ni	^{63}Cu	^{67}Zn	^{71}Ga	^{73}Ge	^{75}As	^{77}Se	^{81}Br	^{83}Kr
23.6	8.9	26.5	6.3	30.6	3.5	17.1	19.1	27.0	3.9
7/2	3/2	3/2	5/2	3/2	9/2	3/2	1/2	3/2	9/2
0.4	?	−0.16	0.15	0.112	−0.2	0.3	–	0.28	0.15
100	1.2	69*‡	4.1	40‡	7.6	100	7.6	49‡	11.5
0.277	6.3×10^{-4}	6.4×10^{-2}	1.2×10^{-4}	5.6×10^{-2}	1.1×10^{-4}	2.5×10^{-2}	5.3×10^{-4}	4.9×10^{-2}	2.2×10^{-4}

^{103}Rh	^{105}Pd	^{109}Ag	^{111}Cd	^{115}In	^{119}Sn	^{121}Sb	^{125}Te	^{127}I	^{129}Xe
3.1	4.1	4.7	21.2	21.9	37.3	23.9	31.6	20.0	27.7
1/2	5/2	1/2	1/2	9/2	1/2	5/2	1/2	5/2	1/2
–	?	–	–	1.16	–	−0.5	–	−0.7	–
100	22	49	13	96	8.6‡	57	7	100	26‡
3.1×10^{-5}	6.2×10^{-5}	4.9×10^{-5}	1.2×10^{-3}	0.332	4.4×10^{-3}	9.2×10^{-2}	2.2×10^{-3}	9.3×10^{-2}	5.6×10^{-3}

^{193}Ir	^{195}Pt	^{197}Au	^{199}Hg	^{205}Tl	^{207}Pb	^{209}Bi	Po	At	Rn
2.0	21.5	1.7	17.8	57.7	20.9	16.1			
3/2	1/2	3/2	1/2	1/2	1/2	9/2			
1.5	–	0.6	–	–	–	−0.4			
62	34	100	17‡	70‡	21*	100			
2.6×10^{-5}	3.4×10^{-3}	2.5×10^{-5}	9.5×10^{-4}	0.14	2.1×10^{-3}	0.137			

^{151}Eu	^{157}Gd	^{159}Tb	^{163}Dy	^{165}Ho	^{167}Er	^{169}Tm	^{171}Yb	^{175}Lu	^{235}U
24.6	4.0	18.2	3.8	17.0	2.5	8.3	17.7	11.3	1.8
5/2	3/2	3/2	5/2	7/2	7/2	1/2	1/2	7/2	7/2
1.16	2	1.3	1.6	2.82	2.83	–	–	5.7	4.1
48	15	100	25	100	23	100	14	97	0.71*
8.7×10^{-2}	5.0×10^{-5}	3.0×10^{-2}	1.6×10^{-4}	0.10	7.1×10^{-5}	5.7×10^{-4}	7.8×10^{-4}	4.8×10^{-2}	8.5×10^{-7}

quadrupole moment Q in units of e x 10^{-24} cm^2, approximate abundance and receptivity relative to the proton are also given. For comparison the free electron has spin $\frac{1}{2}$ and a receptivity of 2.8×10^8 since its magnetic moment is 660 times larger than that of the proton. Its resonant frequency would be ~65 600 MHz in the same field, though in practice lower frequencies are used.

spin states is then:

$$-\frac{m\mu}{I}\mathbf{B_0} \quad \text{or individually} \quad -\mu\mathbf{B_0}, \; -\frac{I-1}{I}\mu\mathbf{B_0}, \; -\frac{I-2}{I}\mu\mathbf{B_0}, \text{etc.}$$

The energy separation between the levels is constant and equals $\mu\mathbf{B_0}/I$. This is shown diagrammatically in Fig. 1.2 for a nucleus with $I = 1$, and positive magnetogyric ratio. The value of m changes sign as it is altered from I to $-I$ and accordingly the contribution of the magnetic moment to total nuclear energy can be either positive or negative, the energy being increased when m is positive. The energy is decreased if the

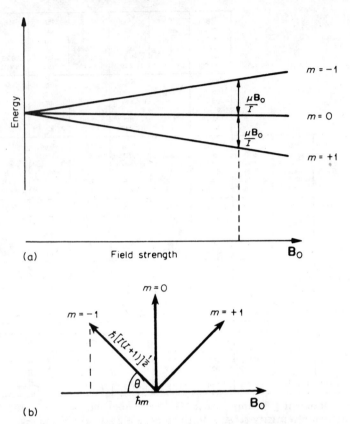

Figure 1.2   (a) The nuclear spin energy for a single nucleus with $I = 1$ (e.g. ^{14}N) plotted as a function of magnetic field $\mathbf{B}_0$. The two degenerate transitions are shown for a particular value of $\mathbf{B}_0$. (b) The alignment of the nuclear vectors relative to $\mathbf{B}_0$ which correspond to each value of m. The vector length is $h[I(I + 1)$ and its z component is $\hbar m$ whence $\cos \theta = m/[I(I + 1)]^{1/2}$.

nuclear magnetic vectors have a component aligned with the applied field in the classical sense. An increase in energy corresponds to aligning the vectors in opposition to the field. Quantum mechanics thus predicts a non-classical situation which can only arise because of the existence of discrete energy states with the high energy states indefinitely stable.

In common with other spectral phenomena, the presence of a series of states of differing energy in an atomic system provides a situation where interaction can take place with electromagnetic radiation of the correct frequency and cause transitions between the energy states. The frequency is obtained from the Bohr relation, namely:

$$hv = \Delta E, \text{the energy separation}$$

For NMR $hv = \mu \mathbf{B_0}/I$

In this case the transition for any nuclear isotope occurs at a single frequency since all the energy separations are equal and transitions are only allowed between adjacent levels (i.e. the selection rule $\Delta m = \pm 1$ operates). The frequency relation is normally written in terms of the magnetogyric ratio (1.1) giving:

$$v = \gamma \mathbf{B_0}/2\pi \tag{1.2}$$

Thus the nucleus can interact with radiation whose frequency depends only upon the applied magnetic field and the nature of the nucleus. Magnetic resonance spectroscopy is unique in that we can choose our spectrometer frequency at will, though within the limitation of available magnetic fields. The values of γ are such that for practical magnets the frequency for nuclei lies in the radio range between a present maximum of 600 megahertz (MHz) and a minimum of a few kilohertz (kHz).

1.3   The source of the NMR signal

The low frequency of nuclear magnetic resonance absorption indicates that the energy separation of the spin states is quite small. Since the nuclei in each of the states are in equilibrium, this suggests that the numbers in the different spin states will be similar, although if there is a Boltzman distribution among the spin states then we can expect more nuclei to reside in the lowest energy states. For a system of spin 1/2 nuclei a Boltzman distribution would give:

$$N_h/N_1 = \exp\left(-\Delta E/kT\right)$$

where N_h and N_1 are the numbers of nuclei in the high and low energy states, respectively, ΔE is the energy separation, k is the Boltzman constant, and T is the absolute temperature. ΔE is given above as $\mu \mathbf{B_0}/I$ which for $I = 1/2$, equals $2\mu \mathbf{B_0}$. Thus:

$$N_h/N_1 = \exp\left(-2\mu \mathbf{B_0}/kT\right)$$

which since $N_h \approx N_1$ can be simplified to:

$$N_h/N_1 = 1 - 2\mu \mathbf{B_0}/kT$$

For hydrogen nuclei in a field of 14 000 gauss (14 kG, 1.4 T, NMR frequency 60 MHz)

$$2\mu\mathbf{B}_0/kT \approx 10^{-5}$$

The excess population in the low energy state is thus extremely small. As far as the overall nuclear magnetism of the sample is concerned the effect of all the nuclei in the high energy state will be cancelled by opposing nuclei in the low energy state, only the small excess number with low energy being able to give rise to an observable magnetic effect, or apparently to absorb radiation.

If $I > 1/2$ one obtains a similar though more complex picture since the excess low energy nuclei do not all have the same value of $m\mu/I$.

It will be noticed that the size of the excess low energy population is proportional to $\mathbf{B}_0$. For this reason the magnetic effect of the nuclei and therefore the intensity of their NMR signal increases as the strength of the magnetic field is increased.

We have so far built up a picture of the nuclei in a sample polarized with or against the magnetic field and lying at an angle θ to it. The total angular momentum (i.e. the length of the vectors of Fig. 1.2) is $[I(I + 1)]^{1/2}$ and the angle θ is then given by:

$$\cos \theta = m/[I(I + 1)]^{1/2}$$

This angle can also be calculated classically by considering the motion of a magnet of moment μ in an applied magnetic field. It is found that the magnet axis becomes inclined to the field axis and wobbles or precesses around it. The magnet thus describes a conical surface around the field axis. The half apex angle of the cone is equal to θ and the angular velocity around the cone is $\gamma\mathbf{B}_0$ so that the frequency of complete rotations is $\gamma\mathbf{B}_0/2\pi$, the nuclear resonant frequency (Fig. 1.3a). This precession is known as the Larmor precession.

For an assembly of nuclei with $I = 1/2$ there are two such precession cones, one for nuclei with $m = +1/2$ and one for $m = -1/2$ and pointing in opposite directions. It is usual however to consider only the precession cone of the excess low energy nuclei, and this is shown in Fig. 1.3b, which represents them as spread evenly over a conical surface and all rotating with the same angular velocity around the magnetic field axis which is made the z axis. Since the excess low energy nuclear spins all have components along the z axis pointing in the same direction, they add to give net magnetization M_z along the z axis. Individual nuclei also have a component μ_{xy} transverse to the field axis in the xy plane. However, because they are arranged evenly around the z axis, these components all average to zero, i.e. $M_x = M_y = 0$. The

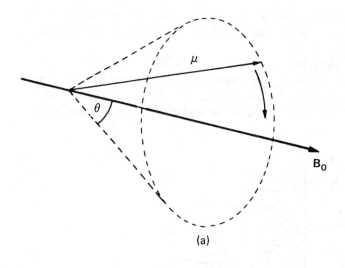

(a)

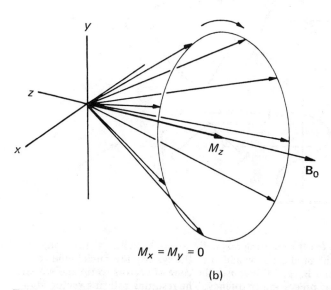

$M_x = M_y = 0$

(b)

Figure 1.3   Freely precessing nuclei in a magnetic field $\mathbf{B_0}$. Larmor
precession of (a) a single nucleus (b) the excess low energy nuclei in a
sample. The nuclear vectors can be regarded as being spread evenly over
a conical surface. They arise from different atoms but are drawn with
the same origin.

magnetism of the system is static and gives rise to no external effects other than a very small, usually undetectable, nuclear paramagnetism due to M_z.

In order to detect a nuclear resonance we have to perturb the system. This is done by applying a sinusoidally oscillating magnetic field along the x axis with frequency $\gamma \mathbf{B}_0/2\pi$ (Fig. 1.4). This can be thought of as stimulating both absorption and emission of energy by the spin system

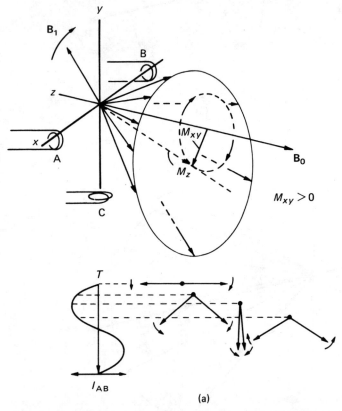

(a)

Figure 1.4   (a) If a rotating magnetic vector $\mathbf{B}_1$ with the same angular velocity as the nuclei is now added to the system, the nuclei tend to precess around $\mathbf{B}_1$ and this causes the cone of vectors to tip and wobble at the nuclear precession frequency. The resulting rotating vector M_{xy} in the xy plane can induce a current in coil C (which is normally placed in the xz plane but is shown below this in the figure for clarity). The lower diagram shows how the vector $\mathbf{B}_1$ can be generated by RF currents I flowing in coils AB. The resulting oscillating field can be resolved into two equal vectors rotating in opposite senses.

(i.e. as stimulating upward and downward spin transitions), but resulting in net absorption of energy, since more spins are in the low energy state and are available to be promoted to the high energy state.

Classically we can analyse the oscillating magnetic field into a super-position of two magnetic vectors rotating in opposite directions. These add at different instants of time to give a zero, positive or negative resultant (Fig. 1.4). The vector $\mathbf{B_1}$ which is rotating in the same sense as the nuclei is stationary relative to them, since we have arranged that it should have the same angular velocity. The nuclei thus precess around $\mathbf{B_1}$ also and the precession cone axis is displaced from the main field axis. Since the nuclear moments do not now all have the same component in the xy plane they no longer cancel in the xy direction and there is resultant magnetization M_{xy} transverse to the main field and rotating at the nuclear precession frequency. The magnetism of the system is no longer static and the rotating vector M_{xy} will induce a radio frequency current in a coil C placed around the sample.

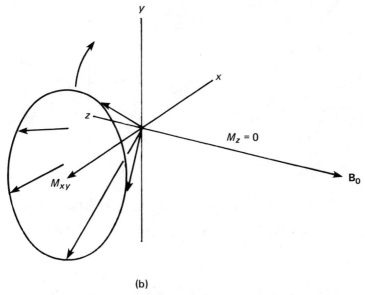

(b)

Figure 1.4   (b) A sufficiently long or powerful $\mathbf{B_1}$ will turn the nuclear precession cone axis into the xy plane and the whole of the nuclear magnetization then contributes to the signal picked up by C (not shown in (b)) and the output is at a maximum. $\mathbf{B_1}$ is thus applied in the form of a pulse and a pulse which has the effect illustrated is known as a $90°$ pulse. The spins follow a spiral path away from the $\mathbf{B_0}$ axis during the pulse.

The arrangement shown in Fig. 1.4 is called the crossed coil arrangement and ensures that C does not pick up any $\mathbf{B_1}$ signal, only that due to the nuclei. If $\mathbf{B_1}$ is of large amplitude then the axis of the precession cone tips quickly and the voltage induced in C increases, reaching a maximum when the nuclear magnets have precessed $90°$ around $\mathbf{B_1}$. When $\mathbf{B_1}$ is cut off, of course this precession stops. In practice it is possible to cause a $90°$ precession in very short times of between 2 and 200 μs (1 $\mu s = 10^{-6}$ s). The coil C then detects the nuclear signal with no interference from $\mathbf{B_1}$ though the signal intensity diminishes to zero as the system returns to equilibrium with $M_{xy} = 0$. An output will be observable in general for between 10 ms and 10 s. Since the signal persists much longer than does the oscillatory pulse which produces $\mathbf{B_1}$, it is possible to dispense with coils A, B and first create $\mathbf{B_1}$ by applying power to C and then detecting the nuclear signal which follows the pulse. This is a single coil spectrometer.

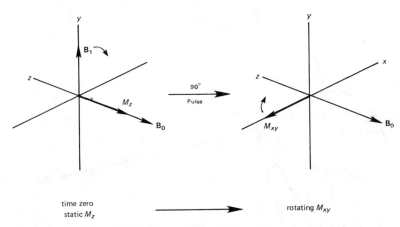

Figure 1.5   A simplified form of Fig. 1.4 in which only the behaviour of the resultant nuclear magnetization is depicted.

If $\mathbf{B_1}$ does not precess at the same frequency as the nuclei then the nuclear precession around $\mathbf{B_1}$ is always changing direction and so M_{xy} can never become significant. It is this feature where the signal is obtained from all the excess low energy nuclei acting in concert and only at a single frequency, which gives to the technique its name of resonance spectroscopy.

1.4   A basic NMR spectrometer

We are now in a position to understand the principles underlying the construction of an NMR spectrometer. The object is to measure the frequency of a nuclear resonance with sufficient accuracy. The instrument (Fig. 1.6) comprises a strong, highly stable magnet in whose gap the sample is placed and surrounded by transmitter–receiver coil C. The magnet may be of three types: permanent, electromagnet or a superconducting (cryo) magnet for the highest field strengths. The field stability is ensured in the first case by placing the magnet in an isothermal enclosure whose temperature is controlled so as to drift not more than 10^{-4} degrees per hour. An extremely stable power supply is used to energize the electromagnet and then an auxiliary coil is used to detect remaining field variations and so to provide correcting adjustments. The superconducting magnet needs no current supply once the field is set up and so is inherently stable, though correcting circuits are still necessary. The magnetic field at the sample also inevitably varies throughout the bulk of the sample (i.e. the field is non-homogeneous) so that the signal frequency is not well defined and a further set of coils, known as shim coils, is placed around the sample in order to counteract these variations or field gradients and render the field as perfectly homogenious as possible. The shim coils are not shown. Remaining inhomogeneities are minimized by spinning the sample tube about its long axis so that the sample molecules experience average fields. Very well defined frequencies, and so excellent resolution of close, narrow resonances is obtained in this way. The $\mathbf{B_1}$ field is produced by a gated (switched input) power amplifier driven by a stable, crystal controlled continuous oscillator. Because the $\mathbf{B_1}$ pulse is very short, its frequency is less well defined than that of the mono-chromatic crystal oscillator and has a bandwidth of $1/t$ Hz (t is the length of the pulse in seconds). It thus does not need to be exactly in resonance with the nuclei and indeed can cause simultaneous precession of nuclei with different frequencies. The nuclear signals are then amplified and detected in a device which compares them with the crystal oscillator output ($\mathbf{B_1}$ carrier) and gives a low frequency, time dependent output containing frequency, phase and amplitude information. This output is digitized and collected in a computer memory for frequency analysis using a Fourier transform program, and the spectrum which results (a spectrum is a function of frequency) can be output to an *XY* recorder and the resonance frequencies listed on a printer.

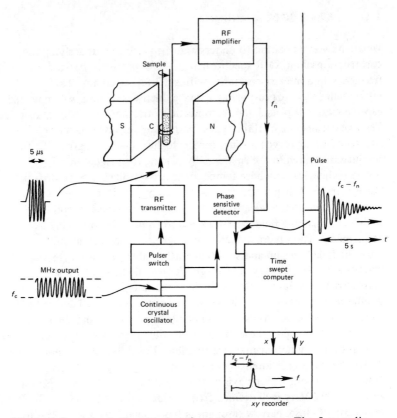

Figure 1.6   A basic Fourier transform spectrometer. The 5 μs radio frequency (RF) pulse tips the nuclei in the sample by $90°$ provided their frequency lies within the bandwidth of the pulse (the pulse switching in effect converts the monochromatic crystal frequency f_c into a band of frequencies of width $1/t$, where t is the pulse length. In this case the bandwidth is 200 000 Hz). The nuclear output signal will be at a frequency f_n close to f_c and the difference frequency $f_c - f_n$ is obtained at the output of the phase sensitive detector. The computer collects the output and then calculates the frequency of resonance relative to f_c. The resonance frequency has limited definition (i.e. it has width) which is related to the time for which the output signal persists. Note that a time dependent output is converted to a frequency dependent output for analysis. Note also the very different time scales for the RF pulse and the output here given the arbitrary lengths of 5 μs and 5 s. The computer and pulser have to be linked in some way to synchronize pulse timing and data collection.

This type of spectrometer is known as a Fourier transform (FT) spectrometer. It is also possible to obtain spectra from the more receptive nuclei using a much simpler system which dispenses with the pulser and computer and produces the recording of the spectrum directly. This is the continuous wave (CW) spectrometer. All early high resolution spectrometers were of this type and indeed the modern FT instruments were developed from these.

2
The Magnetic Field at the Nucleus

2.1   Effects due to the molecule

So far we have shown that a single isotope gives rise to a single nuclear
magnetic resonance in an applied magnetic field. This really would be
of little interest to the chemist except for the fact that the magnetic
field at the nucleus is never equal to the applied field, but depends in
many ways upon the structure of the molecule in which the atom
carrying the nucleus resides.

The most obvious source of perturbation of the field is that which
occurs directly through space due to nuclear magnets in other atoms in
the molecule. In solids this interaction results in considerable broadening
of the resonance which obscures much information. In liquids, on the
other hand, where the molecules are rotating rapidly and randomly,
these fields are averaged to zero, and the lines are narrow and show
much structure. For this reason chemists have been concerned primarily
with liquid samples, and these will be the main preoccupation of this
book. We will nevertheless see later that it has now proved possible to
treat solids so as to diminish these through-space effects and obtain
narrowed lines.

Since the magnetic nuclei do not perturb the field at the nucleus we
have therefore to consider the effect that the electrons in the molecule
may have. We will concern ourselves only with diamagnetic molecules
at this stage and will defer till later discussion of paramagnetic
molecules possessing an unpaired electron. When an atom or molecule
is placed in a magnetic field the field induces motion of the electron
cloud such that a secondary magnetic field is set up. We can think of
the electrons as forming a current loop as in Fig. 2.1 centred on a

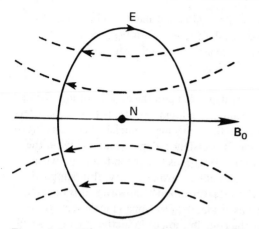

Figure 2.1   The motion of the electronic cloud E around the nucleus N gives rise to a magnetic field, shown by dashed lines, which opposes $\mathbf{B_0}$ at the nucleus.

positively charged atomic nucleus. The secondary field produced by this current loop opposes the main field at the nucleus and so reduces the nuclear frequency. The magnitude of the electronic current is proportional to $\mathbf{B_0}$ and we say that the nucleus is screened (or shielded) from the applied field by its electrons. This concept is introduced into equation (1.2) relating field and nuclear frequency by the inclusion of a screening constant σ.

$$\nu = \frac{\gamma \mathbf{B_0}}{2\pi}(1 - \sigma) \tag{2.1}$$

σ is a small dimensionless quantity and is usually recorded in parts per million, ppm. The screening effect is related to the mechanism which gives rise to the diamagnetism of materials and is called diamagnetic screening.

The magnitude of the effect also depends upon the density of electrons in the current loop. This is a maximum for a free atom where the electrons can circulate freely, but in a molecule the free circulation around an individual nucleus is hindered by the bonding and by the presence of other positive centres, so that the screening is reduced and the nuclear frequency increased. Since this mechanism reduces the diamagnetic screening it is known as a paramagnetic effect. This is unfortunately a misleading term and it must be emphasized that it does not imply the presence of unpaired electrons or indeed that there is an actual paramagnetic current. As used here it merely indicates that there are two contributions to σ, the diamagnetic term σ_d and the paramagnetic term σ_p and that these are opposite in sign. Thus:

$$\sigma = \sigma_d + \sigma_p \tag{2.2}$$

Since the magnitude of σ_d depends upon the density of circulating electrons, it is common to find in the literature discussion of the effect of inductive electron drifts on the screening of nuclei. The screening of protons in organic molecules, for instance, depends markedly on the substituents, and good linear correlations have been found between screening constants and substituent electronegativity, thus supporting the presence of an inductive effect. Currently, however, it is believed that most of these variations originate in the long range effects to be described below and that the contribution of inductive effects is small at least for σ bonded systems.

The magnitude of the paramagnetic contribution σ_p is zero for ions with spherically symmetrical s states but is substantial for atoms, particularly the heavier ones with many electrons in the outer orbitals, which are involved in chemical bonding. It is determined by several factors. (i) The inverse of the energy separations ΔE between ground and excited electronic states of the molecule. This means that correlations are found between screening constants and the frequency of absorption lines in the visible and ultra violet. (ii) The relative electron densities in the various p orbitals involved in bonding, i.e. upon the degree of asymmetry in electron distribution near the nucleus. (iii) The value of $\langle 1/r^3 \rangle$, the average inverse cube distance from the nucleus to the orbitals concerned. In the case of hydrogen, for which there are few electrons to contribute to the screening, and for which ΔE is large, σ_d and σ_p are both small and we observe only a small change in σ among its compounds, most of which fall within a range of 20×10^{-6} or 20 ppm. In the case of elements of higher atomic number, ΔE tends to be smaller and more electrons are present, so that, while both σ_d and σ_p increase, σ_p increases disproportionately and dominates the screening. Thus changes in σ_p probably account for a major part of the screening changes observed for boron in its compounds (a range of 200 ppm), and σ_p almost certainly predominates for fluorine where the range is 1000 ppm, or for thallium where it is 4800 ppm. The changes observed for the proton are thus unusually small.

The observable changes in screening do not increase continuously with atomic number but exhibit a periodicity, increasing with atomic number along each period but then falling again at the start of the next.

The screening range increases down each group but also falls markedly between the element at the foot of a group and the one at the head of the next. This is a consequence of the $\langle 1/r^3 \rangle$ term which exhibits similar periodicity.

The changes observed in screening among the compounds of one element depend primarily upon factors (i) and (ii) above, which means that they are determined by such factors as bond angles and bond order.

The effect of bond angles upon screening is well demonstrated by the phosphorus resonances of some phosphines. ^{31}P screening decreases by 335 ppm between phosphine, PH_3, with bond angles of $93.7°$, and trifluorophosphine, PF_3, with bond angles of $104°$. More strikingly, the screening decreases by 125 ppm between trimethyl phosphine, PMe_3, and tri-t-butyl phosphine, PBu_3^t, owing to the increase in bond angle caused by steric crowding in the t-butyl compound.

The effect of changes in bond order upon screening is exemplified by the fluorine resonances of the pair of diatomic molecules hydrogen fluoride, HF, and fluorine, F_2. The former possesses considerable ionicity in its bond while the latter is highly covalent. F_2 thus should have a large paramagnetic contribution to screening while HF should have little, and as expected HF is 630 ppm more highly screened than is F_2. Perversely, rather than being still more highly screened, the fully ionic fluoride ion, F^-, falls between F_2 and HF, but this probably reflects involvement of the fluoride ion in ion-solvent interactions, so that it is not strictly a free ion. However, in the case of gallium compounds the gallium resonance of the gallium (I) ion, Ga^+, does appear at higher applied magnetic field than any other gallium resonance so far reported. It is the most highly screened gallium nucleus and so has the least paramagnetic contribution to σ.

Usually the contributions to σ_d and σ_p for a nucleus are considered only for the electrons immediately neighbouring, or local to, that nucleus. More distant electrons give rise to long range effects on both σ_p and σ_d which are large but cancel to make only a small net contribution to σ. It is therefore more convenient to separate the long range effects into net contributions from different, quite localised, parts of the rest of the molecule. Two types of contribution to screening can be recognized and though they are small they are of particular importance for the proton resonance.

2.1.1   Neighbour anisotropy effects

We have already mentioned that in liquid samples, owing to the rapid

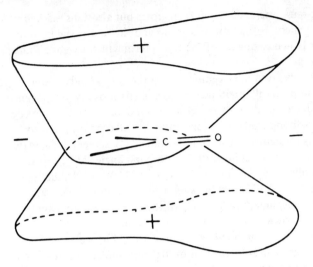

Figure 2.2   Screened and descreened volumes of space around a carbonyl bond. The sign + indicates that a nucleus in the space indicated would be more highly screened. The magnitude of the screening falls off with increasing distance from the group and is zero in the surface of the solid figure.

and random motion of the molecules, the magnetic fields at each nucleus owing to all other magnetic dipoles average to zero. This is only true if the magnet (e.g. a nucleus) has the same dipole strength whatever the orientation of the molecule relative to field direction. If the source of magnetism is anisotropic and the dipole strength varies with orientation in the applied field then a finite magnetic field appears at the nucleus.

Such anisotropic magnets are formed in the chemical bonds in the molecule, since the bonding electrons support different current circulation at different orientations of the bond axis to the field. The result is that nuclei in some parts of the space near a bond are descreened while in other parts the screening is increased. Figs. 2.2 and 2.3 show the way screening varies around some bonds.

A special case of anisotropic screening where the source of the anisotropy is clearly evident occurs in aromatic compounds and in acetylenes or nitriles, which exhibit what is called ring current anisotropy. The benzene structure for instance can support a large electronic ring current around the conjugated π bond system when the plane of the ring is transverse to the field axis but very little when the

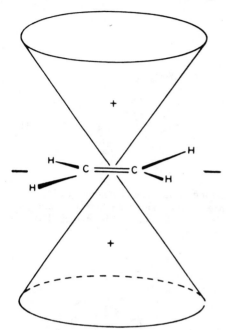

Figure 2.3   Screened and descreened volumes of space around a carbon—carbon double bond. The significance of the signs is the same as in Fig. 2.2 The cone axis is perpendicular to the plane containing the carbon and hydrogen atoms.

ring lies parallel to the field axis. This results in large average descreening of benzene protons since the average secondary magnetic field, which must oppose the applied field within the current loop, acts to increase the field outside the loop in the region of the benzene protons (Fig. 2.4). Similarly the completely filled double π system of a triple bond can be regarded as supporting a ring current. The protons of acetylene however in contrast to those of benzene are further screened by the ring current anisotropy since they lie on the ring current axis (Fig. 2.5).

We are now in a position to understand qualitatively the changes in screening constants $\Delta\sigma$ observed for protons in a number of hydro-carbons* (Fig. 2.6). The anisotropies, including that of the carbon-carbon single bond, play a considerable part in determining the screening constants.

---

* The absolute value of σ is obtained only with difficulty.

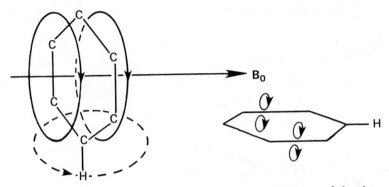

Figure 2.4   Ring current descreening in benzene. The area of the ring current loops due to the π-electrons is much smaller when the plane of the ring lies along the field axis and the reaction field is smaller. The reaction field is shown by a dashed line.

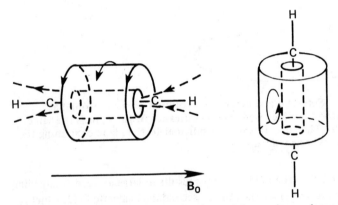

Figure 2.5   Ring current screening in acetylene where a large ring current is sustained around the C–C bond axis when this axis coincides with the applied field direction. The electron cloud is depicted as a cylinder.

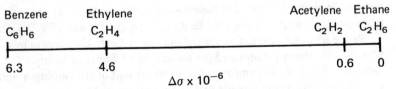

Figure 2.6   Changes in screening constants $\Delta\sigma$ for protons in some hydrocarbons with ethane arbitrarily taken as zero. Following convention the most highly screened protons are placed on the right so that increased $\Delta\sigma$ corresponds to reduced screening.

The position of acetylene tends to emphasize the small effect of inductive electron drifts. The protons of acetylene are acidic and carry the least electron density yet they are highly screened due to the ring current anisotropy of the triple bond.

2.1.2   Through-space electric field effects

Molecules which contain electric dipoles or point charges possess an electric field whose direction is fixed relative to the rest of the molecule. Such electric fields can perturb the molecular orbitals by causing electron drifts at the nuclei in the bond directions and by altering the electronic symmetry. It has been shown that the screening σ_E due to such electric fields is given by:

$$\sigma_E = -AE_z - BE^2 \tag{2.3}$$

where A and B are constants, $A \gg B$, E_z is the electric field along a bond to the atom whose nuclear screening we require and E is the maximum electric field at the atom. The first term produces an increase in screening if the field causes an electron drift from the bond onto the atom and a decrease if the drift is away from the atom. The second term leads always to descreening. It is only important for proton screening in the solvation complexes of highly charged ions where E can be very large, though it is of greater importance for the nuclei of the heavier elements.

The electric field is of course attenuated with increasing distance. It is an intramolecular effect since the effect of external fields, for which the BE^2 term can be neglected, averages to zero as the molecule tumbles and E continually reverses direction along the bond.

The descreening of protons which occurs in many organic compounds containing electronegative substituents X, probably occurs because of the electric field set up by the polar CX bond. This will also increase with X electronegativity and produce a similar result to an inductive electron drift.

Some typical changes in screening constants among such compounds are illustrated in Fig. 2.7 which is an extended version of Fig. 2.6. Notice how the screening is reduced as the distance between the hydrogen and the polar bond is decreased, HCC:O $>$ HC.O or as the number of polar bonds is increased, $CH_2Cl_2 > CHCl_3$.

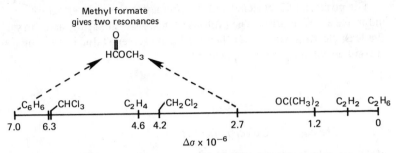

Figure 2.7   Changes in screening constants $\Delta\sigma$ for the protons in hydrocarbons and some molecules containing electric dipolar bonds. Note that increasing the number of carbon—chlorine bonds in the halomethanes results in a progressive decrease in σ. All but one of the compounds has been chosen with chemically indistinguishable protons and these give singlet resonances. Compounds with chemically distinguishable protons such as methyl formate give a resonance for each type of proton.

2.2   Effects due to unpaired electrons

The electron (spin = 1/2) has a very large magnetic moment, and if, for instance, paramagnetic transition metal ions are present in the molecule large effects are observed. The NMR signal of the nuclei present may be undetectable but under certain circumstances, when the lifetime of the individual electron in each spin state is short, so that its through-space effect averages to near zero, NMR spectra can be observed. The screening constants measured in such systems, however, cover a very much larger range than is normal for the nucleus and this arises because the electronic spins can be apparently delocalized throughout a molecule and appear at, or contact, nuclei. The large resonance displacements which result are known as contact shifts and the ligands in certain transition metal ion complexes exhibit proton contact shifts indicating several hundred ppm changes in σ. In addition, if the magnetic moment of the ion is anisotropic, one gets a through-space contribution to the contact interaction similar to the neighbour anisotropy effect and this is called a pseudo-contact shift.

Organic molecules containing polar groups form weak complexes with octahedral organometallic lanthanoid complexes, which have extra bonding orbitals available. These have an anisotropic moment and so cause pseudo-contact shifts throughout the organic molecule. This can result in a wider spread of its spectrum and so simplify its interpretation, and if the molecule is rigid, may allow its conformation to be calculated since the magnitudes and directions of the shifts depends upon the position of the nucleus relative to the polar group.

2.3   The chemical shift

So far we have talked in terms of changes in screening of nuclei. It is, however, more usual to use the term 'chemical shift, rather than the cumbersome phrase 'the relative change in screening brought about by changes in chemical environment'. Thus if we have two nuclei in different environments with screening constants σ_1 and σ_2 then the two nuclear frequencies in a given magnetic field $\mathbf{B_0}$ are:

$$\nu_1 = \frac{\gamma \mathbf{B_0}}{2\pi} (1 - \sigma_1) \tag{2.4a}$$

$$\nu_2 = \frac{\gamma \mathbf{B_0}}{2\pi} (1 - \sigma_2) \tag{2.4b}$$

whence

$$\nu_1 - \nu_2 = \frac{\gamma \mathbf{B_0}}{2\pi} (\sigma_2 - \sigma_1) \tag{2.5}$$

We cannot measure the absolute value of $\mathbf{B_0}$ accurately enough for this relation to be of use, so we eliminate field from the equation by dividing through by ν_1 (equation 2.4a). This gives us the frequency change as a fraction of ν_1:

$$\frac{\nu_1 - \nu_2}{\nu_1} = \frac{\sigma_2 - \sigma_1}{1 - \sigma_1}$$

which since $\sigma_1 \ll 1$ reduces to:

$$\frac{\nu_1 - \nu_2}{\nu_1} = \sigma_2 - \sigma_1 \tag{2.6}$$

Thus the fractional frequency change is the same as the difference in screening in the two nuclear environments. This is called the chemical shift and is given the symbol δ. Its value is expressed in parts per million (ppm). It can be determined with high accuracy since it is possible to detect a frequency difference of 0.1 Hz in 100 MHz (0.001 ppm) for the narrow lines obtained with spin $\frac{1}{2}$ nuclei; even less in favourable cases.

The chemical shift is calculated as follows: the frequency separation between the protons in benzene and methylene chloride is found to be 124.2 Hz at 60 MHz operating frequency ($B_0 = 14.1$ kilogauss (kG) or 1.41 T), then the chemical shift is:

$$\delta = \frac{124.2}{60\,000\,000} \times 10^6 \text{ ppm} = 2.07 \text{ ppm}$$

Or, more easily remembered, it is the shift in Hz divided by the operating frequency in MHz. The frequency separation will of course be different in a spectrometer operating at a different frequency, though δ will be the same.

Because the chemical shift measurement is a relative term it is only possible to define a chemical shift scale for a nucleus if some substance is arbitrarily chosen as a standard and its δ set equal to zero. Thus in Fig. 2.7 ethane is the standard and the scale in units of $\Delta\sigma \times 10^6$ is also a ppm chemical shift (δ) scale.

The usual standard for proton (^1H), carbon (^{13}C) or silicon (^{29}Si) spectra is tetramethylsilane, $(CH_3)_4Si$, usually abbreviated to TMS. This substance gives a narrow singlet resonance in each case (the protons must be decoupled when observing ^{13}C or ^{29}Si — see later) which is well separated from most of the resonances likely to be observed; it is miscible with most organic solvents; it is inert in most systems, and being highly volatile, can easily be removed after measurements have been made. In the case of ^1H and ^{13}C spectroscopy the resonances of interest come predominantly from nuclei which are less screened than is TMS. The TMS signal is taken as origin and shifts, δ, are measured as being increasingly descreened. Thus the ^1H δ for benzene is about 7.37 ppm in deutero-chloroform solution.

It is usual in recording spectra to depict the descreened region to the left-hand side of the spectrum with TMS to the right. The frequency then increases to the left of TMS since the magnetic fields at descreened nuclei are apparently higher and the nuclear precession frequency is higher.

For historical reasons however, this region is very commonly referred to as 'low field', the aptness of this name being apparent from equation 2.1. Both the names 'low field' and 'high frequency' are met in practice, the latter being the most logical, since in a fixed field instrument it is indeed the frequencies which change. The older name though does explain the apparently eccentric way in which the shifts are displayed. This is summarized in Fig. 2.8. Because we have chosen our standard arbitrarily we also find that we have introduced sign into

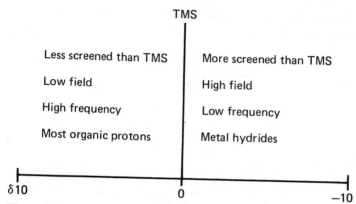

Figure 2.8   Summary of proton chemical shift scales.

the δ scale. Thus in ^{1}H spectroscopy all those protons high field of TMS (low frequency) have negative δ values.

It is of course possible to use subsidiary standards which are referred in turn to TMS, and $(CH_3)_4N^+$ or $(CH_3)_3Si(CH_2)_3COOH$ are often used for ^{1}H spectroscopy in aqueous solutions.

The conventions adopted for other nuclei are less firm. The shifts are usually large so that it is not quite so important to be able to compare different workers' results with high accuracy and the standard substance is often chosen according to the dictates of convenience. The standard is assigned 0 ppm and the δ scales are then as in Fig. 2.8. A dilute aqueous salt solution is often used as standard for groups 1, 2, 3 and 7; $^7Li^+_{aqu}$ for lithium, $^{27}Al(H_2O)_6^{3+}$ for aluminium and $^{35}Cl^-_{aqu}$ for chlorine, for instance. Some much used references are $(CH_3O)_3B$ and $(CH_3CH_2)_2O \rightarrow BF_3$ for ^{11}B spectroscopy, nitromethane CH_3NO_2 or nitrate ion NO_3^- for ^{14}N and ^{15}N spectroscopy, H_2O for ^{17}O spectroscopy, 85% orthophosphoric acid, H_3PO_4, or occasionally P_4O_6 for ^{31}P spectroscopy and the refrigerant $CFCl_3$ is commonly used as standard or as solvent and standard for ^{19}F work. In this last case the chemical shift scale was often called the ϕ scale in the past. Other standards for ^{19}F spectroscopy are hexafluoro benzene C_6F_6 or trifluoroacetic acid CF_3COOH. Some shift scales are summarized in Fig. 2.9.

When reading the literature it is well also to remember that the symbol δ is used extensively as shorthand for the words 'chemical shift', quite independently of standard, and that in older work the sign convention may be reversed, while for protons a τ (tau) scale is common where $\tau = 10 - \delta$.

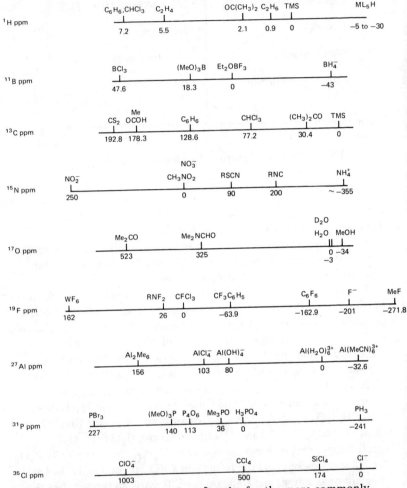

Figure 2.9   Some chemical shift or δ scales for the more commonly used NMR nuclei with the shifts of some substances indicated. TMS is tetramethylsilane. In ^{1}H spectroscopy the hydride resonance is found markedly to high field of TMS. In the case of carbon spectroscopy, the resonances are spread out over a much wider range than the corresponding proton resonances though they fall in much the same order. Carbon atoms carrying no hydrogen can however be observed, as for instance the carbonyl in acetic acid at 178.3 ppm. In nitrogen spectroscopy, the NO_3^- ion resonates close to methyl nitrate at -2.6 ppm.

3
Internuclear Spin–Spin Coupling

3.1   The mutual effects of nuclear magnets on resonance positions

The Brownian motion in liquid samples averages the through-space
effect of nuclear magnets to zero. However, in solutions of $POCl_2 F$,
for example, the phosphorus nucleus gives two resonances whose
separation does not depend upon the magnetic field strength.* This
suggests that the two resonances correspond to the two spin orientations
of the fluorine nucleus and that the nuclei *are* able to sense one anothers
magnetic fields. Theoretical considerations indicate that the interaction
occurs via the bonding electrons. The contact between one nucleus and
its *s* electrons perturbs the electronic orbitals around the atom and so
carries information about the nuclear energy to other nearby nuclei in
the molecule and perturbs their nuclear frequency. The effect is mutual
and in the molecule above both the fluorine ($I = \frac{1}{2}$) and the phosphorus
($I = \frac{1}{2}$) resonances are split into doublets of equal Hz separation. The
magnitude of the effect for a particular pair of nuclei depends on the
following factors. (i) The nature of the bonding system, i.e. upon the
number and bond order of the bonds intervening between the nuclei
and upon the angles between the bonds. The interaction is not usually
observed over more than five or six bonds and tends to be attenuated as
the number of bonds increases though many cases are known where
coupling over two bonds is less than coupling over three bonds. (ii) The
magnetic moments of the two nuclei and is directly proportional to the
product $\gamma_A \gamma_B$ where γ_A and γ_B are the magnetogyric ratios of the
interacting nuclei. (iii) The valence *s* electron density at the nucleus

* The chlorine nuclei ($I = 3/2$) have no effect. This is explained on p. 74.

and therefore upon the s character of the bonding orbitals. This factor also means that the interaction increases periodically as the atomic number of either or both nuclei is increased in the same way as does the chemical shift range.

The magnitude of the coupling interaction is measured in Hz since it is the same at all magnetic fields. It is called the coupling constant and is given the symbol J; its magnitude is very variable and values have been reported from 0.05 Hz up to several thousand Hz. The value of J gives information about the bonding system but this is obscured by the contribution of γ_A and γ_B to J. For this reason correlations between the bonding system and spin–spin coupling often use the reduced coupling constant, K, which is equal to $4\pi^2 J/(h\gamma_A\gamma_B)$.

It is important to understand that coupling constants can be either positive or negative and that the frequency of one nucleus may be either increased or decreased by a particular orientation of a coupled nucleus, the sign depending upon the bonding system and upon the sign of the product $\gamma_A\gamma_B$.

Considerable data are available upon the magnitudes of interproton spin coupling constants from the mass of data accumulated for organic compounds. Interproton coupling is usually (though not always) largest between geminal protons, H.C.H., and depends upon the angle between the two carbon–hydrogen bonds. J_{gem} is typically 12 Hz in saturated systems. J falls rapidly as the number of intervening bonds is increased, being 7 to 8 Hz for vicinal protons (H.C.C.H.) and near zero across four or more single bonds. The same rules apply if oxygen or nitrogen forms part of the coupling path, and methoxy protons H_3COCHR_2 do not usually show resolvable coupling to the rest of the molecule though alcoholic or amino protons may do so to vicinal protons in, for example, $HOCH_3$. On the other hand, coupling may be enhanced if there is an unsaturated bond in the coupling path, due to a σ–π configuration interaction and may be resolved over up to as many as nine bonds, e.g. $^9J(H{-}H) = 0.4$ Hz between the hydrocarbon protons in $H_3C(C \equiv C)_3CH_2OH$. In saturated molecules a planar zig-zag configuration of the bonds may also lead to resolvable coupling over four or five single bonds. Note the use of the superscript 9 in the acetylene example to indicate the number of bonds over which the interaction occurs.

Karplus has calculated the values of the vicinal interproton coupling constants and shown that these depend upon the dihedral angle ϕ between the carbon–hydrogen bonds (Fig. 3.1). Two curves are shown to emphasize that the magnitude of coupling depends also upon the

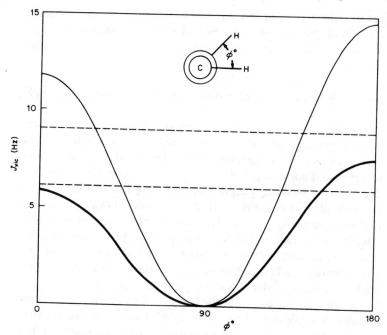

Figure 3.1   Karplus curves relating the dihedral angle ϕ in a HC–CH fragment and the vicinal proton–proton coupling constant. The inset diagram shows a view along the carbon–carbon bond. Two curves are shown relating to differently substituted fragments and are differentiated by heaviness of line. The dotted lines show the typical range of values obtained when a group can rotate freely giving rise to an averaged J_{vic}. (After Jackman and Sternhell *NMR Spectroscopy in Organic Chemistry*.)

nature of the other substituents on the carbon, i.e. upon their electronegativity, their orientation, the hybridization at the carbon, upon the bond angles other than the dihedral angle and upon the bond lengths. For instance, the vicinal coupling in ethyl derivatives decreases with increasing substituent electronegativity. J_{vic} is a rotational average of a Karplus curve because the methyl group rotates freely, and is 6.9 Hz in ethyl fluoride and 8.4 Hz in ethyl lithium. The curves cannot therefore be used to measure ϕ accurately but can often be used to distinguish a correct structure from a number of possibilities or to follow changes in conformation in closely related compounds. An example of this is given in Chapter 9, p. 202 and the validity of the Karplus curve is demonstrated in Fig. 6.3, p. 137, though before we consider these we must find out how to recognize multiplicity which arises from spin coupling and how to determine J. Karplus-type relationships apply also to most other nuclei.

3.2   The appearance of multiplets arising from spin—spin coupling

The appearance of these multiplets is very characteristic and contains much information additional to that gained from the chemical shifts of each resonance. For this reason we intend to go into their analysis in some detail if not in depth. The simplest case to consider is the effect that a single chemically unique nucleus of $I = \frac{1}{2}$ has on other nuclei in the molecule that are sufficiently closely bonded. In half the molecules in the sample the spin of our nucleus N will be oriented in the same direction as the field and all the other nuclei in these molecules will have corresponding resonance positions. In the remainder of the molecules the spin of N will be opposed to the field and all the other nuclei in this half of the sample will resonate at slightly different frequencies to their fellows in the first half. Thus when observing the sample as a whole each of the nuclei coupled to N gives rise to two lines. The line intensities appear equal since the populations of N in its two states only differ by about 1 in 10^5 which is not detectable. We say that N splits the other resonances into 1:1 doublets. Because the z component of magnetization of N has the same magnitude in both spin states the lines are equally displaced from the chemical shift positions of each nucleus which are therefore at the centres of the doublets.

Let us in illustration consider the molecule $CHCl_2 CH_2 Cl$ and its proton resonance. This contains two sorts of hydrogen with the $CHCl_2$ proton resonating to low field of the $CH_2 Cl$ protons due to the greater electric field effect of two geminal chlorine—carbon bonds. The two $CH_2 Cl$ protons have the same frequency since rotation around the carbon—carbon bond averages their environments and makes them chemically and magnetically equivalent. We say they are isochronous. They are mutually spin coupled, but, because they are isochronous give rise to a singlet resonance in the absence of other coupling. We can state as a rule that isochronous protons always resonate as if they were a unit and give a singlet resonance unless coupled to other nuclei. This is why the substances depicted in Fig. 2.7 give rise to singlets despite the presence of coupling between the protons. We will see later that this is a consequence of second-order effects.

In the present example, however, the CH_2Cl resonance is split into a 1:1 doublet because of coupling to the non-isochronous $CHCl_2$ proton. Equally, since the coupling interaction is mutual, the $CHCl_2$ proton is split by the two CH_2Cl protons, though the splitting pattern is more complex. We can discover the shape of the $CHCl_2$ multiplet in several ways.

(i) By an arrow diagram (Fig. 3.2). In some molecules both the CH_2Cl spins will oppose the field, in others both spins will lie with the field while in the remainder they will be oriented in opposite directions. The $CHCl_2$ protons in the sample can each experience one of three different perturbations and their resonance will be split into a triplet. Since the CH_2Cl spins can be paired in opposition in two different ways there will be twice as many molecules with them in this state as there are with them in each of the other two. The $CHCl_2$ resonance will therefore appear as a 1:2:1 triplet with the spacing between the lines the same as that of the CH_2Cl 1:1 doublet. An actual spectrum is shown in Fig. 3.3.

Note that the line intensities are not exactly as predicted by this simple first-order theory due to more complex effects which we will

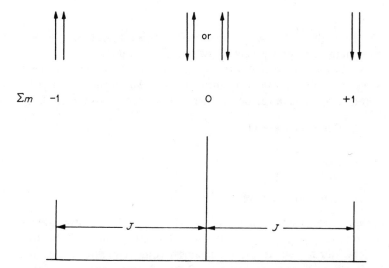

Figure 3.2   A stick diagram demonstrating the splitting due to two spin 1/2 nuclei. When $\Sigma m = 0$ there is no perturbation of the coupled resonance so that the centre line corresponds to the chemical shift position. This holds for all multiplets with an odd number of lines. The spacing J between the lines corresponds to a change in Σm of unity.

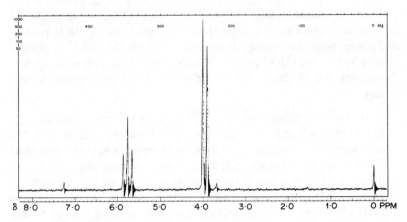

Figure 3.3   60 MHz proton spectrum of $CH_2ClCHCl_2$. The highest
field resonance is due to the protons of TMS. The compound was
dissolved in deuterochloroform ($\sim$ 7% solution) and the $\frac{1}{2}$% or so of
protons in the solvent appears at 7.3 ppm. The resonances are
asymmetric with a ringing pattern to high field of each. This indicates
that they were obtained in the CW mode. (Reproduced by permission
of Varian International AG.)

discuss shortly. Note also that the total multiplet intensity is proportional
to the number of protons giving rise to each multiplet.

(ii) We can also work out the multiplicity by considering the possible
values of the total magnetic quantum number Σm of the two CH_2Cl
protons. $I = \frac{1}{2}$, and m can be $\pm\frac{1}{2}$, therefore for two protons (Fig. 3.2):

$$\Sigma m = +\tfrac{1}{2} + \tfrac{1}{2} = +1$$

or $\quad \Sigma m = +\tfrac{1}{2} - \tfrac{1}{2}$
$\qquad\qquad\qquad = 0$
$\quad$ or $\quad -\tfrac{1}{2} + \tfrac{1}{2}$

or $\quad \Sigma m = -\tfrac{1}{2} - \tfrac{1}{2} = -1$

Therefore we have three lines. Methods (i) and (ii) are equivalent, but
method (ii) is particularly useful when considering multiplets due to
nuclei with $I > \frac{1}{2}$ where arrow diagrams become rather difficult to write
down clearly. Note that when $\Sigma m = 0$ there is no perturbation of the
chemical shift of the coupled group so that the centre of the spin
multiplet corresponds to the chemical shift of the group.

Next let us consider the very commonly encountered pattern given
by the ethyl group CH_3CH_2-. The isochronous pair of CH_2 protons are

usually found low field of the CH_3 protons and are spin coupled to them. The CH_3 protons therefore resonate as a 1:2:1 triplet. The splitting of the CH_2X resonance caused by the CH_3 group can be found from Fig. 3.4, and is a 1:3:3:1 quartet. A typical ethyl group spectrum is shown in Fig. 3.5.

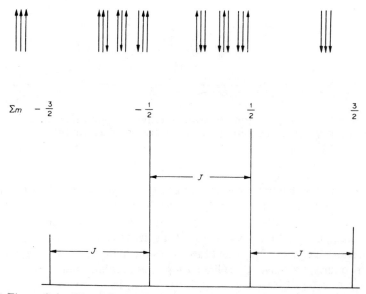

Figure 3.4   The splitting due to three spin 1/2 nuclei. There is no line which corresponds to $\Sigma m = 0$. The multiplet is however arranged symmetrically about the $\Sigma m = 0$ position so that the centre of the multiplet corresponds to the chemical shift position. This rule holds for all multiplets with an even number of lines.

We have done enough now to formulate a simple rule for splitting due to groups of spin $\frac{1}{2}$ nuclei. Thus the number of lines due to coupling to n equivalent spin $\frac{1}{2}$ nuclei is $n + 1$. The intensities of the lines are given by the binomial coefficients of $(a + 1)^n$ or by Pascal's triangle which can be built up as required. This is shown in Fig. 3.6. A new line of the triangle is started by writing a 1 under and to the left of the 1 in the previous line and then continued by adding adjacent figures from the old line in pairs and writing down the sum as shown. The multiplicity enables us to count the number of spin $\frac{1}{2}$ nuclei in a group and the intensity rule enables us to check our assignment in complex cases where doubt may exist, since the outer components of

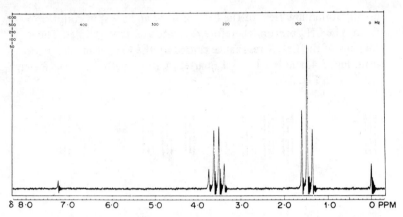

Figure 3.5   60 MHz proton spectrum of ethyl chloride CH_3CH_2Cl. Also a CW spectrum. (Reproduced by permission of Varian International AG.)

resonances coupled to large groups of nuclei (e.g. the CH of $(CH_3)_2CH\cdot$) may be too weak to observe in a given spectrum.

Coupling to nuclei with $I > \frac{1}{2}$ leads to different relative intensities and multiplicities. In the case of a single nucleus the total number of spin states is equal to $2I + 1$ and this equals the multiplicity. If $I = \frac{1}{2}$ we get two lines, $I = 1$ gives three lines, $I = \frac{3}{2}$ gives four lines and so on.

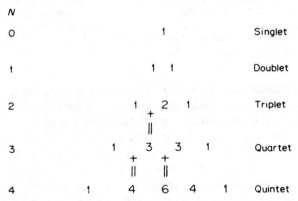

Figure 3.6   Pascal's triangle can be used to estimate the intensities of the lines resulting from coupling to different numbers, N, of equivalent spin 1/2 nuclei. The figures in each line are obtained by adding adjacent pairs of figures in the line above.

The spin populations of each state are virtually equal and so the lines are all of equal intensity and of equal spacing (Fig. 3.7a–d).

Splitting due to multiple combinations of $I > \frac{1}{2}$ nuclei is much less common but a few examples have been recorded. Fig. 3.7 illustrates the origin of the pattern commonly encountered when obtaining ^{1}H spectra in the solvent deutero-6-acetone, $(CD_3)_2 CO$. In practice there will always be a small amount of hydrogen present in these molecules and some of the methyl groups will be $CD_2 H-$ groups. The proton sees two equivalent deuterons with $I = 1$. The maximum total Σm is $1 + 1 = 2$. $\Delta m = \pm 1$ and there are therefore 5 spin states and the proton resonance will be a quintet. In order to determine the line intensities we have to determine the number of ways each value of Σm can be obtained. This is shown in Table 3.1 and indicates relative intensities of 1:2:3:2:1, a distribution which differs from the simple binomial. Table 3.2 illustrates the calculation for two ^{11}B nuclei ($I = 3/2$).

Table 3.1   Line intensities for coupling to two nuclei with $I = 1$

Σm	Possible spin combinations	Number of spin combinations
2	(+1 +1)	1
1	(+1 0) (0 +1)	2
0	(+1 −1) (0 0) (−1 +1)	3
−1	(−1 0) (0 −1)	2
−2	(−1 −1)	1

Table 3.2   Line intensities for coupling to two nuclei with $I = 3/2$)

Σm	Possible spin combinations	Number of spin combinations
3	$(+\frac{3}{2} +\frac{3}{2})$	1
2	$(+\frac{1}{2} +\frac{3}{2}) (+\frac{3}{2} +\frac{1}{2})$	2
1	$(+\frac{1}{2} +\frac{1}{2}) (+\frac{3}{2} -\frac{1}{2}) (-\frac{1}{2} +\frac{3}{2})$	3
0	$(+\frac{3}{2} -\frac{3}{2}) (-\frac{3}{2} +\frac{3}{2}) (+\frac{1}{2} -\frac{1}{2}) (-\frac{1}{2} +\frac{1}{2})$	4
−1	$(-\frac{1}{2} -\frac{1}{2}) (-\frac{3}{2} +\frac{1}{2}) (+\frac{1}{2} -\frac{3}{2})$	3
−2	$(-\frac{1}{2} -\frac{3}{2}) (-\frac{3}{2} -\frac{1}{2})$	2
−3	$(-\frac{3}{2} -\frac{3}{2})$	1

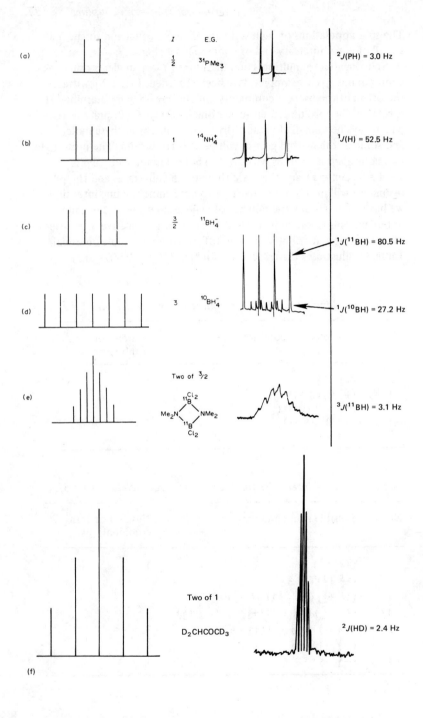

(a) I E.G. $\frac{1}{2}$ $^{31}PMe_3$ $^2J(PH) = 3.0$ Hz

(b) 1 $^{14}NH_4^+$ $^1J(H) = 52.5$ Hz

(c) $\frac{3}{2}$ $^{11}BH_4^-$ $^1J(^{11}BH) = 80.5$ Hz

(d) 3 $^{10}BH_4^-$ $^1J(^{10}BH) = 27.2$ Hz

(e) Two of $\frac{3}{2}$

$$Me_2N \underset{\underset{Cl_2}{B}}{\overset{\overset{Cl_2}{\underset{11}{B}}}{}} NMe_2$$

$^3J(^{11}BH) = 3.1$ Hz

(f) Two of 1

$D_2CHCOCD_3$

$^2J(HD) = 2.4$ Hz

While Table 3.3 gives that for three deuterons which have the same maximum Σm. A third type of pattern is obtained.

The rule given for spin $\frac{1}{2}$ nuclei can be generalized to include groups of nuclei of any I. The number of lines observed for coupling to n equivalent nuclei of spin I is $2nI + 1$.

Table 3.3   Line intensities for coupling to three, nuclei with I = 1

Σm	Possible spin combinations	Number of spin combinations
3	(+1 +1 +1)	1
2	(+1 +1 0) (+1 0 +1) (0 +1 +1)	3
1	(+1 0 0) (0 +1 0) (0 0 +1) (−1 +1 +1) (+1 −1 +1) (+1 +1 −1)	6
0	(0 0 0) (0 +1 −1) (+1 0 −1) (+1 −1 0) (0 −1 +1) (−1 0 +1) (−1 +1 0)	7
−1	(−1 0 0) (0 −1 0) (0 0 −1) (+1 −1 −1) (−1 +1 −1) (−1 −1 +1)	6
−2	(−1 −1 0) (−1 0 −1) (0 −1 −1)	3
−1	(−1 −1 −1)	1

More complex coupling situations also arise where a nucleus may be coupled simultaneously to chemically different groups of nuclei of the same or different isotopes or species. The patterns are found by building up spectra, introducing the interactions with each group of nuclei one at a time. Thus Fig. 3.8 shows how a group M coupled to two

Figure 3.7   Multiplets observed in proton spectra due to coupling to nuclei with various spin quantum numbers. (a)–(d) single nuclei. Examples are given of the proton spectra of trimethylphosphine, of the ammonium ion and of the borohydride anion. Boron contains two isotopes ^{11}B ($I = \frac{3}{2}$) and ^{10}B ($I = 3$) and splitting due to both sorts of boron is observed. The coupling constant to ^{10}B is smaller than that to ^{11}B since the latter has a much larger magnetogyric ratio. (e) Shows the pattern for coupling equally to two ^{11}B nuclei. The ^{10}B multiplet in this case is not observable and leads only to line broadening. Coupling to nitrogen or chlorine is not observed. (f) shows the commonly encountered pattern for coupling equally to two ^2H nuclei, in a deuterated solvent with a small proportion of hydrogen present — deutero acetone.

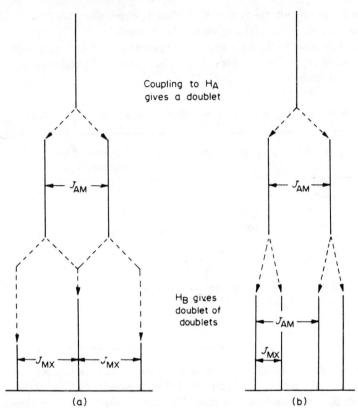

Figure 3.8   Splitting of the H_M protons of $Z_2CH_A-C(H_M)_2-CH_XY_2$ due to coupling to H_A and H_X: (a) $J(A-M) = J(X-M)$, the centre lines overlap and the multiplet is a 1 : 2 : 1 triplet just as if H_M were coupled to a CH_2 group; (b) $J(A-M) \neq J(A-M)$ and we get a doublet of doublets from which both $J(A-M)$ and $J(X-M)$ can be measured.

chemically different spin $\frac{1}{2}$ nuclei A and X is split first by $J(A-M)$ into a doublet and shows that each doublet line is further split by $J(M-X)$. If $J(A-M) = J(A-X)$ a 1:2:1 triplet is obtained, but if $J(A-M) \neq J(A-X)$ then a doublet of doublets with all lines of equal amplitude arises. This can be distinguished from a ^{11}B coupling because the line separations are irregular and of course the preparative chemist is usually aware whether or not there should be boron in his compound.

In analysing such multiplets it always has to be born in mind that overlap of lines may occur so that fewer than the theoretical number of lines are seen and the intensities are unusual. Such a case is illustrated in Fig. 3.9a for coupling to two equivalent protons and one boron

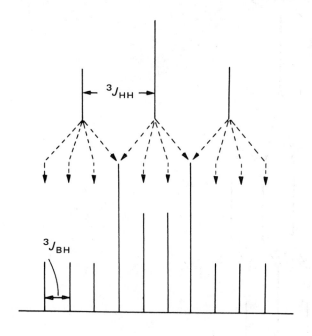

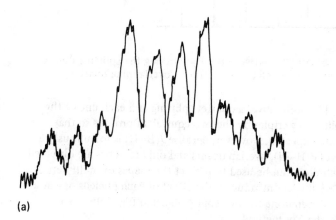

(a)

Figure 3.9   (a) Proton spectrum of the methyl group of $CH_3NH_2BF_3$.
Overlap of lines occurs because $^3J(H-H) = 3 \times {}^3J(^{11}B-H)$. The
superscripts to J refer to the number of bonds between the coupled
nuclei. The methyl protons are coupled resolvably only to boron and
the NH_2 protons. A typical trace is shown below. Coupling to ^{10}B leads
to line broadening.

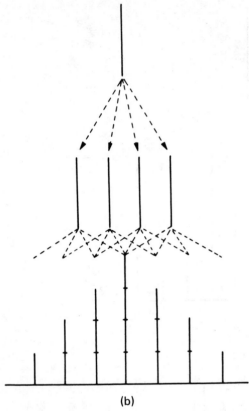

(b)

Figure 3.9   (b) An alternative way of predicting the splitting due to two equivalent spin $\frac{3}{2}$ nuclei as a quartet of overlapping quartets.

nucleus ^{11}B. The boron gives a quartet splitting and each line of the quartet is split into a triplet by the two equivalent protons so that twelve lines are expected. However, because $J(B-H)$ is fortuitously a sub-multiple of $J(H-H)$, overlap occurs and only ten lines are observed. The same technique can be used to predict the shapes of multiplets due to several $I > \frac{1}{2}$ nuclei, introducing the effect of each nucleus one at a time. This has been done for two spin $\frac{3}{2}$ nuclei in Fig. 3.9b as an alternative to the Σm method.

3.3   Spin–spin coupling satellites

We would normally consider the spectrum of methane as being a singlet.

In doing this we are of course thinking only of the molecule $^{12}C^{1}H_4$ and are ignoring the 1.1% of $^{13}C^{1}H_4$ which contains the magnetically active ^{13}C isotope with $I = \frac{1}{2}$. If we looked carefully in the base line we would find a doublet with $J = 125$ Hz centred approximately on the intense singlet due to the main component. These two small lines are termed spin satellites and, while weak, can often be used to obtain extra information about otherwise symmetrical molecules. For example, the molecule $(CF_3S)_3N$ has a singlet fluorine resonance with satellites due to molecules $^{13}CF_3SN(S^{12}CF_3)_2$. The fluorine in the $^{13}CF_3$ group is no longer isochronous with the $^{12}CF_3$ fluorine and the two sorts of fluorine atom can now exhibit spin coupling. As a result the satellites are split into septets by the other six fluorine nuclei bonded to ^{12}C (Fig. 3.10). This, together with the empirical formula, proves the presence of three chemically equivalent CF_3 groups. Note the magnitude of the fluorine–fluorine coupling constants which are often larger than proton–proton coupling constants over the same number of bonds.

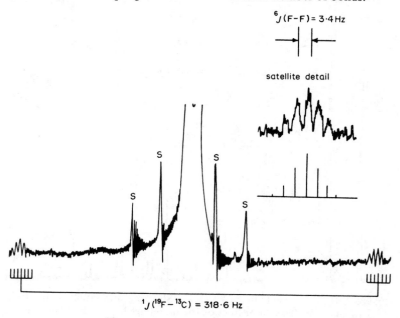

Figure 3.10   The ^{19}F spectrum of $(CF_3S)_3N$ showing the satellites due to 3.3 % of $(^{13}CF_3S)N(^{12}CF_3S)_2$. The fluorine on ^{13}C is split into a septet by long range coupling with the fluorine on ^{12}C, $^6J(F–F) =$ 3.4 Hz, while these latter are mutually split into a quartet. This is lost beneath the singlet due to the all ^{12}C molecule. The lines marked S are spinning sidebands — see p. 134.

The alteration in resonance position caused by the coupling interaction, in this case with ^{13}C, is often described as introducing an effective chemical shift since it results in the observation of spin coupling interactions which could not be seen between the otherwise equivalent nuclei.

A second example is the spectrum of $W_2O_2F_9^-$ (Fig. 3.11). This consists of a doublet of intensity 8 and a nonet of intensity 1. The nine fluorine atoms can thus be divided into an isochronous set of eight and one unique atom. There are in addition however spin satellite lines due to coupling to the 14.28% of ^{183}W which has a spin $I = \frac{1}{2}$. These lines will originate from the ions $^{183}W^{184}WO_2F_9^-$ since only 2% of the molecules will contain two ^{183}W atoms and their resonance will be much weaker. Each of the lines of the intense doublet has two ^{183}W satellites, each of which is further split into a 1:4:6:4:1 quintet. This pattern must arise from coupling to four fluorine atoms. We can therefore conclude that we have four of the eight isochronous fluorine

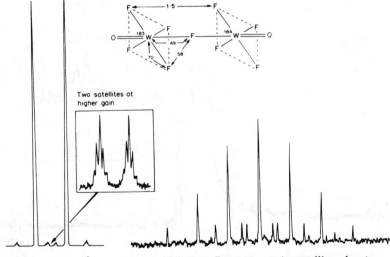

Figure 3.11 ^{19}F spectrum of $W_2O_2F_9^-$ showing spin satellites due to 14.28% of ^{183}W. The outer lines of the nonet are lost in the base-line noise and the student should confirm that the intensity ratios of the observed lines correspond to those expected for the inner seven of the nonet rather than to those expected for a septet. The arrows around the formula indicate the various coupling interactions in Hz. The single fluorine nonet is recorded at higher gain. (After McFarlane, Noble and Winfield (1971) *J. Chem. Soc. (A)*, 948, with permission.)

atoms associated with the ^{183}W atom and therefore split into a satellite doublet and then further coupled to the remaining four which are equally associated with the ^{184}W atom. This provides considerable confirmatory evidence that the structure is $OWF_4 \cdot F \cdot WF_4O$ with a fluorine atom bridging the tungsten atoms.

3.4   Second-order effects

The rules so far discussed apply to spectra of nuclei of the same species where the chemical shifts or the effective chemical shifts are large compared with the coupling constants, or to coupling between nuclei of different species where the frequency separation of lines is invariably large. A nomenclature has been adopted for these cases in which the chemically non-equivalent sets of spins are labelled with letters from the alphabet, choosing letters that are well separated in the alphabetic sequence to signify large chemical shift separation. Thus $CH_2ClCHCl_2$ is an A_2X system, CH_3CH_2R is an A_3X_2 system, and CH_3CH_2F is an A_3M_2X system. Their spectra are called first order.

We have already seen in the examples that the line intensities in proton spectra exhibiting interproton coupling often do not correspond exactly to those predicted by the first-order rules and these distortions increase as the interproton chemical shift is reduced. The spectra are said to become second order and to signify this and the fact that the chemical shifts between the coupled nuclei are relatively small, the spins are labelled with letters close together in the alphabet. Thus, for example, two coupled protons resonating close together are given the letters AB and an ethyl group in $(CH_3CH_2)_3Ga$, where the methyl and methylene protons resonate close together, is described as an A_3B_2 grouping. Mixed systems are also possible and a commonly encountered one is the three spin ABX grouping where two nuclei resonate close together and a third is well shifted or is of a different nuclear species.

Second-order spectra arise when the frequency separation between multiplets due to different equivalent sets of nuclei is similar in magnitude to the coupling constant between them; under these circumstances the effects due to spin coupling and chemical shift have similar energy and become intermingled, leading to alterations in relative line intensities and in line positions. Because it is the ratio between the frequency separation and J which is important, chemical shifts are always expressed in Hz and not in ppm in this context. The Hz separation is obtained by multiplying the chemical shift, δ, by the spectrometer operating frequency and is written $\nu_0\delta$. The perturbation of the spectra from the first-order appearance is then a function of the ratio $\nu_0\delta/J$ and is different for spectrometers operating at different frequencies. If a high enough frequency is used, many second-order spectra approach their first-order limit in appearance and this is one of the advantages of high-field instrumentation.

We will consider the simplest possible system with two spin $\frac{1}{2}$ nuclei, i.e. the AB system. When the chemical shift between them is large then we see two doublets. A typical arrangement with $J = 10$ Hz and $\nu_0\delta = 200$ Hz is shown in Fig. 3.12a. If we reduce the chemical shift progressively to zero we can imagine the two doublets approaching one another until they coincide. However we know that an isolated pair of equivalent nuclei give rise to a singlet and the problem is how can two doublets collapse to give a singlet. If the coupling constant remains at 10 Hz why do we not get a doublet A_2 spectrum?

The behaviour of the multiplets can be predicted using a quantum mechanical argument. The system can have any one of four energy states. These are characterized by the spin orientation of the two nuclei. The wave functions of the two spin states are normally written α for $I = +\frac{1}{2}$ and β for $I = -\frac{1}{2}$. There are four such spin states with the wave functions $\alpha\alpha$, $\alpha\beta$, $\beta\alpha$ and $\beta\beta$, where the first symbol in each pair refers to the state of the A nucleus and the second symbol to the state of the B nucleus. The energies of the states $\alpha\alpha$ and $\beta\beta$ can be calculated straight forwardly but the two states $\alpha\beta$ and $\beta\alpha$ have the same total spin angular momentum and it is found that the quantum mechanical equations can only be solved for two linear combinations of $\alpha\beta$ with $\beta\alpha$. This is described as a mixing of the states and means that none of the observed transitions corresponds to a pure A or a pure B transition. The form of the wave functions and the energy levels derived are shown below. C_1 and C_2 are constants, ν_A and ν_B are the A and B nuclear frequencies in the absence of coupling and $\nu_0\delta = |\nu_A - \nu_B|$

No.	Wave function	Energy level (Hz)
1	$\alpha\alpha$	$\frac{1}{2}(\nu_A + \nu_B) + \frac{1}{4}J$
2	$C_1(\alpha\beta) + C_2(\beta\alpha)$	$\frac{1}{2}[(\nu_0\delta)^2 + J^2]^{1/2} - \frac{1}{4}J$
3	$-C_2(\alpha\beta) + C_1(\beta\alpha)$	$-\frac{1}{2}[(\nu_0\delta)^2 + J^2]^{1/2} - \frac{1}{4}J$
4	$\beta\beta$	$-\frac{1}{2}(\nu_A + \nu_B) + \frac{1}{4}J$

The transition energies are the differences between four pairs of energy states, 3–4, 2–4, 1–3, and 1–2, each transition involving a mixed

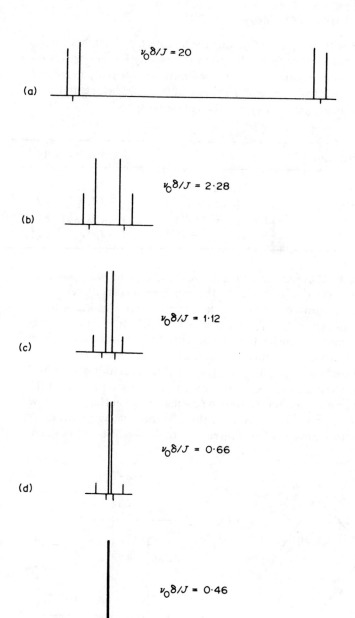

Figure 3.12   AB quartets for several values of the ratio $v_0\delta/J$. The small markers under the base-line represent the true A and B chemical shift.

energy level. Because of the mixing the transition probabilities are no longer equal as in the first-order case and intensity is transferred from lines in the outer parts of the total multiplet into the central region. The transition energies relative to the centre of the multiplet, i.e. to the mean frequency $\frac{1}{2}(\nu_A + \nu_B)$, and the intensities are:

	Transition	Energy (Hz)	Relative intensity
a	$3 \rightarrow 1$	$+\frac{1}{2}J + \frac{1}{2}[(\nu_0\delta)^2 + J^2]^{1/2}$	$1 - J/[(\nu_0\delta)^2 + J^2]^{1/2}$
b	$4 \rightarrow 2$	$-\frac{1}{2}J + \frac{1}{2}[(\nu_0\delta)^2 + J^2]^{1/2}$	$1 + J/[(\nu_0\delta)^2 + J^2]^{1/2}$
c	$2 \rightarrow 1$	$+\frac{1}{2}J - \frac{1}{2}[(\nu_0\delta)^2 + J^2]^{1/2}$	$1 + J/[(\nu_0\delta)^2 + J^2]^{1/2}$
d	$4 \rightarrow 3$	$-\frac{1}{2}J - \frac{1}{2}[(\nu_0\delta)^2 + J^2]^{1/2}$	$1 - J/[(\nu_0\delta)^2 + J^2]^{1/2}$

There are thus four lines as in the AX spectrum but with perturbed intensities. The line positions and the corresponding energy level diagram are shown in Fig. 3.13. The energy levels are marked with the appropriate spin state and the transitions which in the first-order case can be regarded as arising from transitions of the A or B nucleus from opposite sides of the figure. The three line separations are $a-b = J$, $c-d = J$, and $b-c = [(\nu_0\delta)^2 + J^2]^{\frac{1}{2}} - |J|$. The separation $a-c$ or $b-d$ which in the first-order case is the same as the separation between the doublet centres, and is therefore the chemical shift in Hz, $\nu_0\delta$, is now simply $[(\nu_0\delta)^2 + J^2]^{\frac{1}{2}}$ and is larger than the true chemical shift. In other words, though $\nu_0\delta$ is reduced to zero the doublet centres never

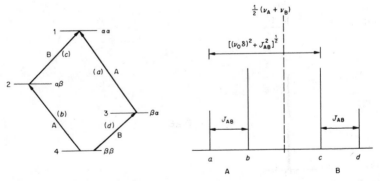

Figure 3.13   The energy level diagram for a system of two spins related to the resulting AB quartet. The spectrum was calculated for $J = 10.0$ Hz, $\nu_0\delta = 28.2$ Hz, i.e. $\nu_0\delta/J = 2.82$.

coincide and are separated by J Hz. The outer lines however have intensity zero at this point while the inner lines are coincident, i.e. we predict a singlet spectrum as is observed. C.f. Fig. 3.12e. Thus arises our rule 'isochronous coupled protons resonate as a unit'.

We can calculate some simple rules for analysing an AB spectrum.

(i) The spectrum contains two intervals equal to J, a–b and c–d.

(ii) The true AB chemical shift $\nu_0\delta$ is found as follows:

$$(a-d)(b-c) = ([(\nu_0\delta)^2 + J^2]^{\frac{1}{2}} + J)([(\nu_0\delta)^2 + J^2]^{\frac{1}{2}} - J)$$

$$= (\nu_0\delta)^2 + J^2 - J^2$$

$$= (\nu_0\delta)^2$$

therefore

$$\nu_0\delta = [(a-d)(b-c)]^{1/2}$$

a–d is the separation between the outermost lines and b–c is the separation between the innermost pair of lines.

(iii) The assignment can be checked against the intensity ratios of the larger and smaller lines. The intensity ratio, stronger/weaker is:

$$(1 + J/[(\nu_0\delta)^2 + J^2]^{1/2})/(1 - J/[(\nu_0\delta)^2 + J^2]^{1/2})$$

which gives:

$$([(\nu_0\delta)^2 + J^2]^{1/2} + J)/([(\nu_0\delta)^2 + J^2]^{1/2} - J)$$

the ratio of the line separations $(a-d)/(b-c)$.

Note that changing the sign of J does not alter the pattern.

Fig. 3.12a–e shows the form of the AB quartet for several values of $\nu_0\delta/J$. The true chemical shift positions are marked below the base-line. It is important to remember that if a multiplet shows signs of being highly second order then both intensities *and* resonance positions are perturbed from their first-order values. A spacing corresponding to J_{AB} remains in AB type spectra since only one coupling interaction exists, but in more complex systems the spacings are combinations of coupling constants. On the other hand, if the intensity perturbation is only slight (Fig. 3.12a) then the line positions are not detectably perturbed. Three examples of actual spectra which contain an AB multiplet are given in Fig. 3.14.

3.4.1   The three spin system

We shall first construct an energy level diagram for the three spin system similar to that of Fig. 3.13 for the AB system (Fig. 3.15). The

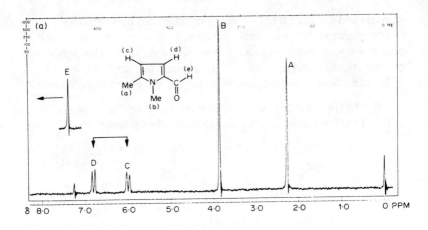

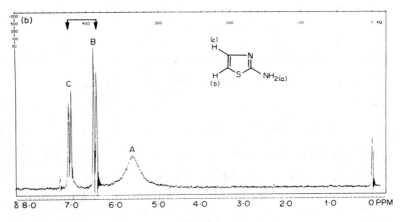

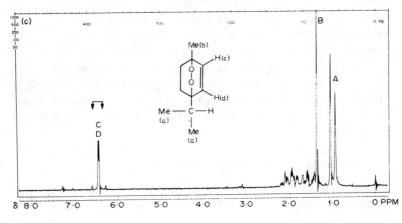

spin orientations are indicated by the signs + or − and are set down in groups of all the possible combinations of three spins, with groups of different total angular momentum placed on different levels. The spins are always written in the order spin 1, spin 2, spin 3 and as laid out the transitions + → − of any one spin form four parallel sides of a cube. Thus the transitions A_1 A_2 A_3 and A_4 occur for a + → − transition of spin 1 in the presence of the spin 2, spin 3 combinations + +, − +, + −, − −.

The cube diagram of Fig. 3.15 is used extensively in analysing three spin spectra. We shall use it to demonstrate how degeneracy arises in NMR spectra and to indicate how the system ABX may be analysed.

First we shall consider how we can obtain the form of the first-order AX_2 spectrum from the cube. If we let spin 1 be nucleus A and spins 2 and 3 be the nuclei X_2, then spins 2 and 3 are isochronous and equally coupled to spin 1. We obtain transitions as follows:

One A transition for X_2 oriented + + (line A_1)   ⎫
Two A transition for X_2 oriented + − (lines A_2 and A_3)   ⎪   giving a
                          or − +   ⎬   1:2:1
(These are now indistinguishable)   ⎪   triplet
One A transition for X_2 oriented − − (line A_4)   ⎭

Two X_2 transitions for A oriented + (lines $B_1 C_1 B_3 C_3$) ⎫ giving a
Two X_2 transitions for A oriented − (lines $B_2 C_2 B_4 C_4$) ⎬ 4:4 doublet

Figure 3.14   60 MHz spectra of some compounds containing AB groupings of protons, in order of decreasing $\nu_0 \delta/J$. The AB quartets are at low field in each case and are bracketed. (a) 1, 5-dimethyl pyrrole-2-aldehyde. E is offset and is observed at 9.38 ppm. Protons (C) and (D) give the AB quartet. (b) 2-aminothiazole. Note the broad line arising from hydrogen on ^{14}N. Protons (B) and (C) give the AB quartet. (c) Ascaridole. Protons (C) and (D) give the AB quartet. Note also the complex second-order spectrum due to the ring methylene protons at ca. 1.9 ppm which also overlap the septet due to the CH proton in the $CHMe_2$ group. This spectrum is highly complex because rotational averaging of the proton positions is not possible and each proton has different coupling constants to each of the others.

In $\overset{H_1}{\underset{H_2}{\diagup}} C \text{——} C \overset{\diagdown H_3}{\underset{\diagdown H_4}{}}$ $^3J(H_1 - H_3) \neq\ ^3J(H_2 - H_3)$

and none of the protons is *magnetically* equivalent. see p. 56

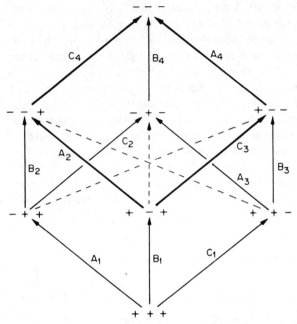

Figure 3.15   An energy level diagram for a three spin $(I = \frac{1}{2})$ system. Each edge of the cube corresponds to one of the twelve possible transitions. The dashed lines indicate combination transitions where all three spins change orientation simultaneously though Δm remains unity.

We see two X_2 transitions rather than four X transitions since the two nuclei resonate as a unit.

The above description of the spectrum shows that the centre A transition and the two X_2 transitions each consist of two coincident transitions, i.e. they are degenerate transitions. This enables us to understand qualitatively why, when we reduce the A–X chemical shift so as to give a second-order AB_2 spectrum in which the line positions are perturbed, we observe an eight line spectrum. The degeneracies are lifted and we can resolve four A transitions and four B_2 transitions. The line positions and intensities calculated for different $\nu_0\delta/J$ are given in Fig. 3.16. A ninth line is depicted for $\nu_0\delta/J = 2$. This is a combination line which corresponds to a combined transition of all three spins such that $\Delta\Sigma m = 1$, e.g. $- + + \rightarrow + - -$. There are three such possible transitions marked by dashed arrows in Fig. 3.15, which may be observed in second-order spectra. An AB_2-like spectrum is shown in Fig. 9.8.

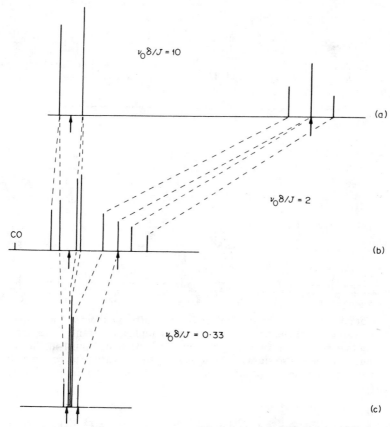

Figure 3.16   Diagram showing how the degenerate lines in an AB_2 spectrum separate as the chemical shift is reduced. In (c) the flanking lines are too weak to be observed. CO is a combination line.

If we make our three nuclei have different chemical shifts with three different coupling constants then in the first-order case, AMX, we have 12 lines. These are represented by the 12 sides of the cube diagram. None of the transitions coincide since none of the + − pair combinations are equivalent (Fig. 3.17).

If we allow the M nucleus to have a similar frequency to the A nucleus then we obtain an ABX spectrum. The AB part is second-order and the close AB coupling leads to second-order perturbation in the X region of the spectrum also. The analysis of the AB part can be accomplished fairly easily if we consider it to be made up of two AB

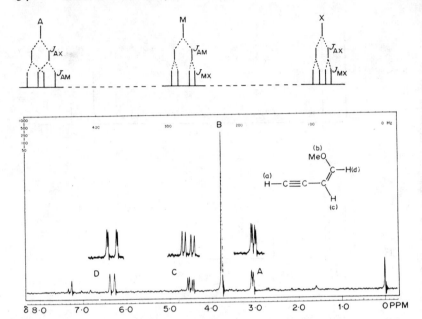

Figure 3.17   Top: The spectral first-order pattern expected for coupling between three nuclei with three different coupling constants (1, 2, and 3 units in this case). An example of an AMX spectrum from 1-methoxy-1-buten-3-yne is also shown. The upper multiplets have been re-run on an expanded scale. (Reproduced by permission of Varian International AG.)

sub-spectra, i.e. one quartet corresponding to X spin = $+\frac{1}{2}$ and one corresponding to X spin = $-\frac{1}{2}$. This is equivalent to separating the cube diagram into two AB diagrams connected by the C transitions. The effective chemical shifts E and E^* used to calculate the line positions and intensities of the AB sub-spectra are, for one (E) $\nu_0\delta_A - \frac{1}{2}J_{AX}$ and $\nu_0\delta_B - \frac{1}{2}J_{BX}$ and for the other (E^*) $\nu_0\delta_A + \frac{1}{2}J_{AX}$ and $\nu_0\delta_B + \frac{1}{2}J_{BX}$. Since $J_{AX} \neq J_{BX}$ the frequency separation of the A and B resonances are not the same in the two AB sub-spectra, the value of $[(\nu_0\delta)^2 + J_{AB}^2]^{1/2}$ is not the same and no line separations corresponding to $J(A-X)$ or $J(B-X)$ can be found in the AB part. This is demonstrated in the scale diagram of Fig. 3.18. Four separations $J(A-B)$ can however be recognized.

The X part, which can arise from the same or a different nuclear species as A and B, consists of four transitions plus two combination lines. Again no spacing corresponding to $J(A-X)$ or $J(B-X)$ exists in

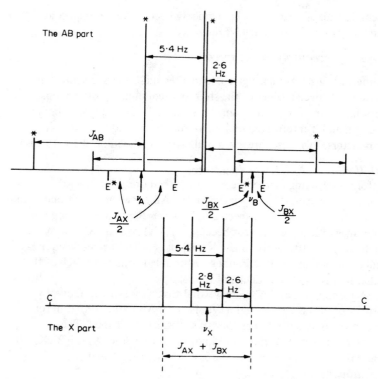

Figure 3.18   Diagram of an ABX spectrum. One AB sub-spectrum is differentiated from the other by the asterisk. The parameters used to calculate line positions and intensities are $|\nu_A - \nu_B| = 10$ Hz, $J(A-B) = 10$ Hz, $J(A-X) = 6$ Hz, and $J(B-X) = 2$ Hz. The positions E, E^* given the effective chemical shifts of each of the AB sub-spectra and are shifted from the true resonance positions ν_A, ν_B by amounts depending on $J(A-X)$ and $J(B-X)$. Because none of E or E^* coincides with the centres of the AB doublets, none of the spacings is equal to $J(A-X)$ (6 Hz) or $J(B-X)$ (2 Hz). Four spacings equal to $J(A-B)$ can however be observed.

the X part though one can be found which corresponds to their sum. The spectrum can be analysed from this and from the effective chemical shifts obtained from the AB part, though there are in general two solutions.

It should be noted that if the sign of $J(B-X)$ is different from that of $J(A-X)$, the line order is altered and the form of the spectrum changes quite drastically. We can thus obtain relative signs of coupling constants in the ABX case. Computers are much used in the analysis of

second-order spectra since these quickly become very complex as the
number of interacting nuclei is increased.

3.4.2   Deceptively simple spectra

Sometimes a set of nuclei give rise to a second-order spectrum which
because of special values of the shifts and coupling constants looks
very like a first-order spectrum. These are called deceptively simple
spectra, and if interpreted on a first-order basis could give the wrong
parameters. Two cases are given in illustration based on the ABX case.

(a) If either $\nu_0 \delta_{AB} = 0$ or $J_{AX} = J_{BX}$
Before proceeding further we have to extend our definition of
equivalent nuclei. If $\nu_0 \delta_{AB} = 0$ then the AB nuclei are isochronous and
we might expect an $A_2 X$ spectrum. However the two nuclei are not
fully magnetically equivalent because $J(A-X) \neq J(B-X)$ and they are
each coupled differently to the X nucleus. For full magnetic equivalence nuclei must be isochronous *and* coupled equally to each of the
other non-isochronous nuclei of the set.

Returning to our ABX case we find that either of the above
situations means that we get a symmetrical AB part and that in the X
region the two central lines overlap giving a 1:2:1 triplet. The
observation of the X triplet need not mean that $J(A-X) = J(B-X)$ while
the AB spectrum may persist despite the fact that A and B are
isochronous.

(b) If $\nu_0 \delta_{AB}$ and $\frac{1}{2}(J(A-X) - J(B-X))/J(A-B)$ are both small
Here we also get an X triplet and the outer lines of the AB sub-spectra
become too small to observe, thus giving the appearance of an $A_2 X$
spectrum, though the spacings do not correspond to any coupling
constant.

3.4.3   Virtual coupling

The typical AMX spectrum consists of twelve lines of equal intensity.
Because the intensities are equal we know it is a first-order spectrum
and that the coupling constants can be measured directly from the line
separations. Now let us see in more detail what happens as we allow the
M resonance to approach the A resonance to give an ABX spectrum
(Fig. 3.19). The perturbation of the X part of the spectrum which
occurs as the AM nuclei approach and become AB can be clearly seen
in the figure. We say that when $J(A-B)/\nu_0 \delta$ is large the system is
strongly coupled.

Now let us consider what would happen to the X spectrum if

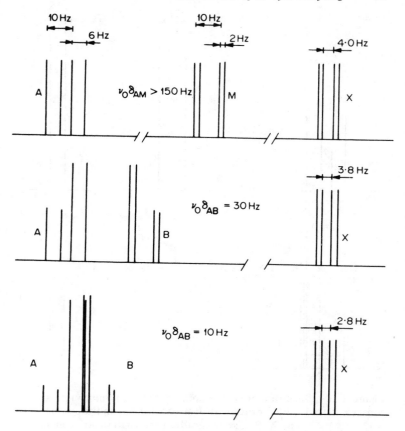

Figure 3.19   Changes which occur in the spectrum of three spin $\frac{1}{2}$ nuclei from pure first-order AMX to second-order ABX. The coupling parameters are the same as in Fig. 3.18.

$J(B–X) = 0$. In the weakly coupled AMX case with $J(M–X) = 0$ the M and X resonances are split into doublets giving a total of eight lines (Fig. 3.20a). However if the AM part becomes strongly coupled (AB) all twelve lines of an ABX spectrum appear (Fig. 3.20b). This is often described as virtual coupling, i.e. X and B are apparently coupled via the strong AB interaction. This often leads to increased complexity in spectra which otherwise might be relatively simple. For instance, the methylene protons of long-chain hydrocarbons often appear as broad bands of overlapping lines rather than as a series of near coincident quintets as might at first be expected.

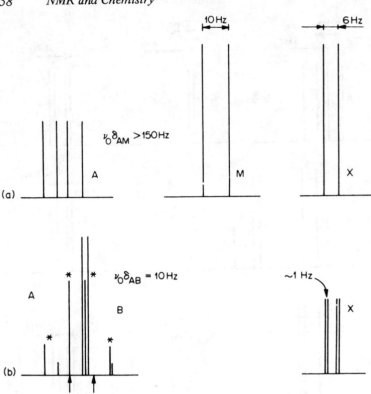

Figure 3.20   Spectrum of a three spin system with one coupling constant zero. (a) First order with $J(M-X) = 0$. (b) In the second-order ABX case with $J(B-X) = 0$, second-order perturbation still occurs in the X part to give four lines. This is described as virtual coupling via the strong AB interaction. The parameters used are $J(A-B) = 10$ Hz, $J(A-X) = 6$ Hz, $J(B-X) = J(M-X) = 0$ Hz, and $|\nu_A - \nu_B| = 10$ Hz.

3.4.4   Spin–spin satellites and second-order effects

Spin satellites may show second-order splitting. For instance, dioxane contains two sets of four isochronous protons (Fig. 3.21). A ^{13}C atom at one position splits the resonance of its attached A protons into a doublet. If we consider the molecules with the ^{13}C nucleus all in one orientation, i.e. those giving rise to one satellite, then these contain two isochronous A nuclei coupled to two isochronous X nuclei resonating at a different frequency. The nucleus A is coupled to X and to X' by different amounts since free rotation is not possible, so that X and X', though isochronous, are not magnetically equivalent. Similarly A and A' are not equivalent. The spectrum is therefore second-order

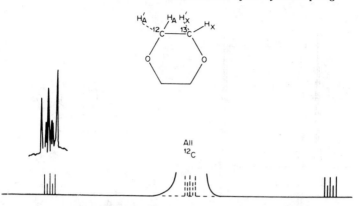

Figure 3.21   The ^{13}C satellite spectrum of dioxane. The ring structure prevents complete rotation of the methylene groups so that $J(A-X)$ and $J(A'-X)$ cannot average to the same value. Protons A and A' are thus not fully equivalent. The inset shows an actual satellite trace. (After Sheppard and Turner (1959) *Proc. Royal Soc.*, A252, 506, with permission.)

even though the AX effective chemical shift is quite large.

Note the use of primes in the above example to differentiate isochronous but magnetically non-equivalent nuclei. In large spin systems the use of primes can become cumbersome and so an alternative nomenclature has been introduced. This would describe the above system as an $[AX]_2$ sub-system.

This example, as does the earlier one involving spin satellites (Fig. 3.10), has a satellite spectrum which is more complicated than the original singlet spectrum, and so gives extra information about the molecule. Where the main spectrum is already second order, that information is already to hand and the problem is how to extract the information, especially if the spectrum is a complex one. In such a case the effective increase in chemical shift for the satellites may well give first-order patterns from which the NMR parameters can be extracted straightforwardly. An example of this approach is given in Fig. 3.22. The spectrum of furan consists of two triplets. This then is a deceptively simple spectrum since the α protons cannot be coupled equally to the two β protons. Under high resolution the central line splits into two components. The values of the four coupling constants can be extracted from the first order patterns of the ^{13}C satellites, A of the α (low field satellite) and B of the β (high field satellite) resonances. Each pattern contains three of the couplings and these were then used to calculate the splittings in the main second-order spectrum.

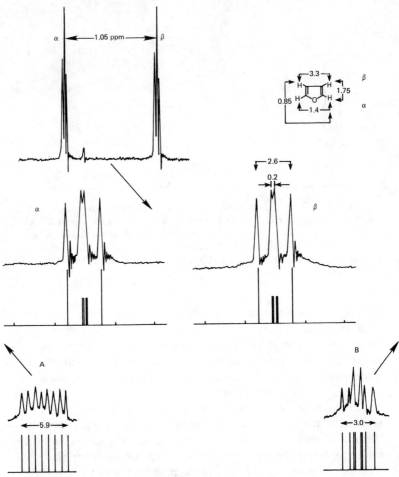

Figure 3.22 ^{1} H NMR spectrum of furan. Coupling constants and splittings are given in Hz. The A satellite is 100.7 Hz to low field of the α multiplet and the B satellite 87.6 Hz to high field of the β multiplet. $^1J(H^{13}C) = 201.4$ Hz and $^1J(H^{13}C) = 175.3$ Hz, respectively. (Reproduced with permission from Reddy and Goldstein (1962) *J. Amer. Chem. Soc.*, **84**, 583.)

4
Nuclear Magnetic Relaxation and Related Phenomena

4.1 Relaxation processes in assemblies of nuclear spins

If we perturb a physical system from its equilibrium condition and then remove the perturbing influence, the system will return to its original equilibrium condition. It does not return instantaneously, however, but takes a finite time to readjust to the changed conditions. The system is said to relax. Relaxation to equilibrium usually occurs exponentially, following a law of the form:

$$(n - n^e)_t = (n - n^e)_0 \exp(-t/T)$$

where $(n - n^e)_t$ is the displacement from the equilibrium value n^e at time t and $(n - n^e)_0$ that at time zero. The relaxation rate can be characterized by a characteristic time T. If T is small, relaxation is fast, whereas if T is large, relaxation is slow.

The concept of the relaxation times appropriate to assemblies of magnetically active nuclei is of high importance to our technique and allows us to understand a considerable number of NMR phenomena. For this reason we intend to cover the subject with some care. We have already noted that in an assembly of spin $\frac{1}{2}$ nuclei the spins in the two energy levels are in equilibrium, a small excess number existing in the low energy level. In Fig. 4.1a these nuclei are shown precessing around a conical surface, and evenly distributed over it. This constitutes an equilibrium condition for our system, with net magnetization M_z in the longitudinal or field axis direction and zero net magnetization M_{xy} transverse to the z axis in the xy plane. This system can be perturbed in two separate ways, either we can change M_z, which means changing the energy of the system, or we can change M_{xy}, which involves no energy

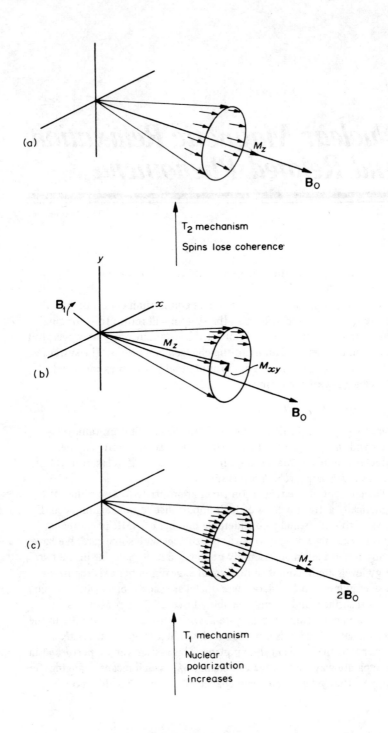

(a)

T_2 mechanism

Spins lose coherence

(b)

(c)

T_1 mechanism

Nuclear
polarization
increases

change. We have already shown that we can make M_{xy} non-zero by introducing the rotating field $\mathbf{B}_1$ (Fig. 1.4) which tips the precession cone axis. This stops when $\mathbf{B}_1$ is switched off and M_{xy} then returns to zero. This occurs because the precession frequencies of the spins are not all the same but cover a range, some being faster and some slower than the nominal resonance frequency. They thus blur out the wobbling precession cone created by $\mathbf{B}_1$ and the spins spiral back to their equilibrium position. We can also say that the spins lose their coherence due to the relaxation process. This takes a finite and often appreciable time since the spread of precession frequencies is not large. This process, affecting the transverse magnetization, is known as transverse relaxation and its characteristic time is given the symbol T_2.

Secondly, we can consider what might happen if we were suddenly to double $\mathbf{B}_0$. This would increase the energy separation between the two spin states and so increase the number of spins expected to remain in the low energy state. In other words the new equilibrium value of longitudinal magnetization M_z is increased. The system will relax to the new value by means of spins undergoing transitions from the upper to the lower energy level. This involves a loss of energy by the system which also requires a finite time. This process, which affects only the longitudinal magnetization, is known as longitudinal relaxation and is given the symbol T_1.

The nuclei in an assembly of atoms are extremely well isolated from their surroundings, so much so that in certain especially pure solid samples values of T_1 of 1000 seconds have been recorded* There is in fact no reason why longitudinal relaxation should take place at all in the absence of stimulating radiation at the nuclear resonant frequency. In liquid samples, however, the values of T_1 for spin $\frac{1}{2}$ nuclei vary typically from about 50 to 0.5 seconds and we have therefore to postulate that fluctuating magnetic fields exist within those samples which cause relaxation. Consideration of the nature of liquids shows that we should expect such fields to exist, since the molecules are undergoing Brownian motion, i.e. diffusing and rotating randomly so that the nuclear magnets in the system are continually moving relative to each other and so produce wildly fluctuating magnetic fields at all

*and in liquids – ^{6}Li in LiCl/D_2O

Figure 4.1   A system of nuclear magnets ($I = \frac{1}{2}$) (a) can be perturbed in two ways, either by altering the field $\mathbf{B}_0$ (c) when the excess population in the lower energy state changes at a rate determined by T_1, or by tipping the precession cone off axis (b) when a return to equilibrium is governed by T_2.

points within the sample. Over the long term these average to zero but at any instant will contain a component of random intensity and phase at the nuclear resonant frequency, and it is this which effects interchange of nuclear energy with the rest of the system and gives rise to the T_1 relaxation mechanism. Since the internal field has different values at each nucleus at each instant of time then they will also have different precession frequencies, which when averaged, gives the spread of frequencies already mentioned so that the Brownian motion also controls the T_2 relaxation mechanism. For this reason T_1 and T_2 are often about equal in liquids. This frequency spread of course means that the resonance frequency is not precisely defined and that the spectral lines have width which is proportional to $1/T_2$.

4.2   Relaxation, Brownian motion and sample viscosity

The internal fluctuating magnetic field which causes relaxation owes its existence to Brownian motion and the time-scale of the motion is one factor which determines its effectiveness. Since Brownian motion is random in character its time-scale is characterized by a somewhat loosely defined term, the correlation time τ_c. This is defined as the time taken on average for a molecule to diffuse a distance equal to its own dimension or to rotate through one radian. τ_c is typically 10^{-11} s in liquids of low viscosity. This corresponds to a frequency of 10^5 MHz. It has been shown that the frequency spectrum of randomly fluctuating fields such as exists within NMR samples is essentially that of 'white' noise and contains all frequencies less than $1/\tau_c$. The field intensity at any frequency, $K(\nu)$, is given by:

$$K(\nu) \propto \frac{2\tau_c}{1 + 4\pi^2 \nu^2 \tau_c^2}$$

This function is plotted in Fig. 4.2a and it will be seen that over the NMR frequency band the relaxation field intensity is constant.

We can find how the value of τ_c is related to the sample viscosity by using the Debye theory of electric dispersion which shows that for a spherical molecule rotating in a liquid, the correlation time and viscosity are related by:

$$\tau_c = \frac{4\pi a^3}{3k} \frac{\eta}{T}$$

where η is the viscosity, T is the temperature and a is the radius of the sphere. Thus if we vary the viscosity of a sample or vary its temperature

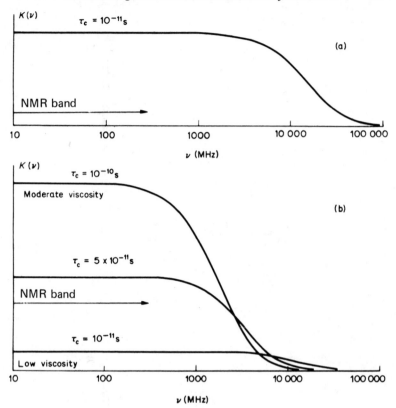

Figure 4.2   Intensity of fluctuations in magnetic fields in a liquid sample due to Brownian motion, as a function of frequency: (a) typical liquid; (b) liquids of different viscosities.

we will alter τ_c. The effect of increasing τ_c is shown in Fig. 4.2b and for the viscosities of liquids normally used as solvents its effect in the NMR band is simply to increase $K(v)$ proportionately, i.e.:

$$K(v) \propto \tau_c \propto \eta/T$$

Thus in order to obtain long relaxation times, T_1 and T_2, and the narrowest resonances, it is necessary to keep the viscosity low. The spectrum of a viscous liquid is compared in Fig. 4.3 with its relatively non-viscous solution to emphasize this point.

It is also worth considering for a moment the relaxation processes in solids. Here there is no Brownian motion so that there is no random relaxing field and T_1 is very long. The magnitude of T_1 is determined

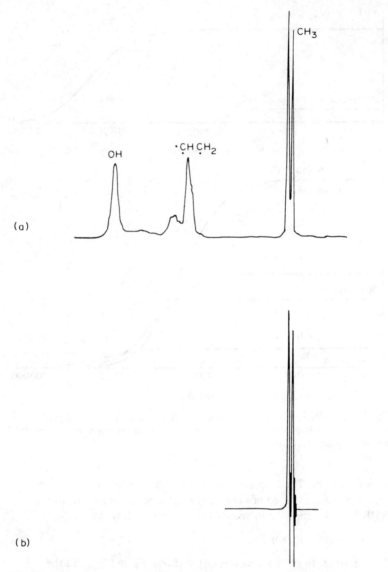

Figure 4.3   Proton spectrum of propylene glycol, $CH_3CHOHCH_2OH$:
(a) neat viscous liquid; (b) 16% solution in deuterochloroform. The
methyl doublet is much better resolved and the well-developed wiggle
pattern shows that the relaxation time is longer. The remaining
resonances are broad due to slow exchange of the OH proton and are
little effected by the viscosity changes – see Section 4.8.

by the concentration of paramagnetic impurities in the solid lattice and for this reason is also known as spin–lattice relaxation. Because of the lack of Brownian motion, neighbouring spins come directly under the influence of each others magnetic fields. This consists of two components, (a) a static one due to the μ_z component of the nuclear magnet along the magnetic field axis and of a magnitude and direction determined by the spin state of the nucleus, and (b) a rotating one due to the transverse field component μ_{xy} of the precessing spin. The rotating component forms a means for the direct interchange of energy between spins and such interchange occurs frequently though with no net change in energy of the nuclear system and therefore no effect on T_1. The lifetime of the individual spin states is shortened drastically by this process and the uncertainty principle dictates that resonances will be broad. T_2 is indeed very short in solids, often in the region of microseconds and line-widths are measured in kilohertz. T_2 is sometimes referred to as spin–spin relaxation.

The static component of the fields of the nuclear magnets determines the line shape. If the nuclei occur in close pairs then for two like, spin $\frac{1}{2}$ nuclei, either will experience one of two magnetic fields depending upon whether the other has the orientation with $m = +\frac{1}{2}$ or $-\frac{1}{2}$. The resonance appears as a broad doublet. If the nuclei occur in close triangular clusters, then individuals experience one of three magnetic fields depending upon whether the spin orientations of the other two give $\Sigma m = +1$, $\Sigma m = 0$ or $\Sigma m = -1$. In this case the resonance appears as a broad 1:2:1 triplet. Weaker interactions with more distant nuclei lead to further multiplicity which is not resolved but contributes further line broadening. The shape of these broadened multiplets can be used to determine internuclear distances which in the case of protons may be difficult to obtain using other techniques.

If we inspect the equation for $K(\nu)$ we will see that the above discussion for liquids concerns only the region where $4\pi^2\nu^2\tau_c^2$ is much less than unity, i.e. the region where

$$2\omega\tau_c \ll 1$$

We call this the region of extreme narrowing, where the correlation time is much shorter than a Larmor period and where $T_1, T_2 \propto 1/\tau_c$. If we have a high nuclear Larmor frequency (high magnetic field) and/or a long correlation time, then

$$2\omega\tau_c \approx 1$$

and new behaviour appears. Now we are at the knee of the curves of

Fig. 4.2 and the spectral density of the noise falls if we increase τ_c and
so the relaxation processes become *less* effective.

4.3   Dipole–dipole relaxation

This is the name given to the part of the nuclear relaxation caused by
the magnetic fields of nearby nuclear dipoles, as discussed above, and is
written T_{1DD}. T_{1DD} is longest when τ_c is short and becomes shorter as
τ_c increases but only while the general rate of motion is sufficient to
ensure that the condition of extreme narrowing is met. When the
motion is slow enough, T_{1DD} increases as τ_c increases and so has a
minimum which depends on ω_0. T_{2DD} behaves like T_{1DD} in the region
of extreme narrowing but when the motion becomes slow compared
with a Larmor period, direct spin–spin energy exchange can occur and
continues to decrease T_{2DD} even though the relaxation field is
decreasing, tending towards the situation outlined for solids (Fig. 4.4).
Knowledge of this behaviour is particularly important for the
spectroscopy of large molecules such as biomolecules or polymers,
which move only slowly in solution and for which line broadening may
be observed in their ^1H or ^{13}C spectra, especially at high field.

The dipole–dipole relaxation times are given by the formulae:

$$1/T_{1DD} = K(\gamma^4/r^6)\{\tau_c/(1 + \omega^2\tau_c^2) + 4\tau_c/(1 + 4\omega^2\tau_c^2)\}$$

$$1/T_{2DD} = K'(\gamma^4/r^6)\{3\tau_c + 5\tau_c/(1 + \omega^2\tau_c^2) + 2\tau_c/(1 + 4\omega^2\tau_c^2)\}$$

The rate of relaxation thus depends strongly upon the magnetogyric
ratio and upon the sixth power of the distance r between the interacting
spins. The mechanism is therefore going to be most important for
nuclei close to hydrogen or fluorine, and specifically for those directly
bonded to them. Other nuclei distant from hydrogen should have rather
longer relaxation times than are found for hydrogenic compounds but
this is found to be true only for spin $\frac{1}{2}$ nuclei. For nuclei with $I > \frac{1}{2}$ the
relaxation times are always shorter than would be expected on the basis
of T_{1DD} alone often by factors as large as 10^8. We therefore have to
consider a second relaxation mechanism for these nuclei.

4.4   Electric quadrupole relaxation

Nuclei with $I > \frac{1}{2}$ possess a quadrupole moment Q which arises because
the distribution of charge in the nucleus is not spherical but ellipsoidal,

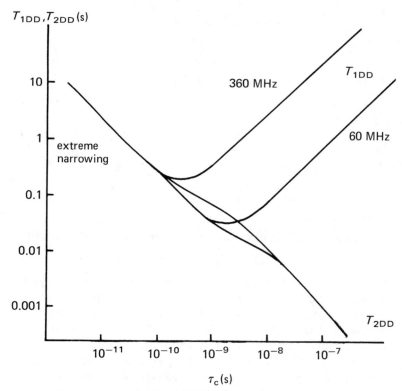

Figure 4.4 Variation of T_{1DD} and T_{2DD} with τ_c for two different spectrometer frequencies. The figures given apply to two protons separated by 160 pm. (After Martin, Depluech and Martin, *Practical NMR Spectroscopy*, John Wiley & Sons Inc., with permission)

i.e. the charge distribution within the nucleus is either slightly flattened (oblate – like the earth at its poles) or slightly elongated (prolate – like a rugby ball). Cross-sections of the charge of two such nuclei are shown in Fig. 4.5 with the departure from spheroidal form much exaggerated. The disposition of the electric quadrupole is also suggested. If the electric fields due to external charges vary across the nucleus then the torque on each dipole component of the quadrupole is different and a net torque is exerted on the nucleus by the electric field as well as by the magnetic fields present. Electric field gradients exist at atomic nuclei due to asymmetries in the spatial arrangement of the bonding electrons. The Brownian tumbling of the molecule causes the direction of the resulting electric quadrupole torque to vary randomly around the

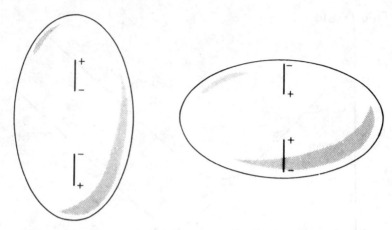

Figure 4.5   Cross-sections of the charge distributions in quadrupolar nuclei.

nucleus in exactly the same way as does the torque due to the magnetic relaxation field. Rotating electric torque components thus exist at the nuclear resonant frequency which can also cause interchange of energy between nucleus and the rest of the system (T_1 mechanism) and randomization of nuclear phase (T_2 mechanism).

The quadrupolar mechanism is a highly effective means of relaxation of many nuclei, and often can be regarded as the sole source of relaxation. Its magnitude depends upon a large number of factors so that the observed relaxation times vary over a very wide range. A simplified form of the quadrupole relaxation equation is given below which emphasizes the importance of nuclear properties I and Q and of the maximum field gradient $-\mathrm{d}_2 V/\mathrm{d}z^2$. T_1 and T_2 are equal in the region of extreme narrowing:

$$\frac{1}{T_1} = \frac{1}{T_2} \propto \frac{(2I+3)Q^2}{I^2(2I-1)} \left(\frac{\mathrm{d}_2 V}{\mathrm{d}z^2}\right)^2 \tau_c$$

Nuclear quadrupole relaxation thus increases rapidly in effectiveness as we move from observing nuclei with small Q to those with large Q, though this is to some extent offset by the factor involving I. This occurs because there is a tendency for large Q to be associated with large I and because the value of $(2I+3)/[I^2(2I-1)]$ falls off rapidly with increasing I. For a given nuclear species the relaxation time is primarily determined by the electric field gradient. This depends mainly upon the electronic symmetry around the nucleus (not upon the symmetry of the molecule as a whole though the two are often linked). A uniform spherical orbital produces zero electric field gradient as does any arrangement of localized charges with cubic symmetry. Thus nuclei of free ions and nuclei of atoms at the centres of strictly regular tetrahedral or octahedral structures formed from a single type of ligand, all possess near zero electric field gradients, long relaxation times and therefore narrow lines. The replacement of a ligand of a regular structure by another, different one then reduces the relaxation time though the effect is often surprisingly small. On the other hand, a distorted octahedron or tetrahedron, even one with all the ligands the same, may have a very short relaxation time and such distortion seems to be a very important source of electric field gradients. In this context of course, it should be remembered that lone pairs of electrons are also ligands. At the other extreme, nuclei in atoms which form a single bond to other groupings have large electric field gradients, short relaxation times and broad, sometimes undetectable lines. The disposition of non-bonding pairs of electrons and of electrons forming π-bonds can however considerably reduce the electric field gradients at such terminal atoms. Table 4.1 contains a number of examples in illustration. For comparison typical natural proton line widths in a perfectly homogeneous field are 0.02 Hz.

Study of the table will indicate what line-widths are to be expected in various situations. Note that in nitrogen compounds the bonding to nitrogen is all important in determining the field gradient so that substitution of H by phenyl in $C_6H_5CH_2NMe_3^+$ produces very little change in line-width though the symmetry of the molecule as a whole changes markedly. The low field gradient at the isocyanide nitrogen is also remarkable.

'Terminal' seems to mean very different things in terms of electric field gradient to chlorine in PCl_3 and nitrogen in MeCN and indicates very different electronic structures around these two atoms. The high field gradient in PCl_3 may suggest that the amount of sp^3 hybridization of the chlorine atoms is quite small, which is consistent with theories that halogens bond principally with their p electrons.

At the same time it must be admitted that there is very little systematic correlation of line-widths with structure and while it is possible to differentiate between atoms in positions of low or high symmetry, little can be said at present about intermediate cases, although in series of related molecules where valid comparisons may be made such as the boron hydrides, parallels are often observed between ^{11}B line-widths (and T_1s) and the chemical shift which suggest that the

Table 4.1 Line-widths of the resonances of selected quadrupolar nuclei

Molecule	Comments	Nuclear resonance line-width (Hz)
^{14}N in:	$f(I, Q) = 0.0012$	
The tetramethylammonium cation Me_4N^+	Strictly regular tetrahedron small N–H coupling resolvable in proton spectrum. $T_1 > 2$ s	0.1
The ammonium cation H_4N^+	Strictly regular tetrahedron Possible broadening due to proton exchange	2
The benzyltrimethylammonium cation $Me_3NCH_2C_6H_5^+$	Symmetry still tetrahedral around N and the phenyl has little influence	~7
The phenylammonium cation $H_3NC_6H_5^+$	One ligand now very different from the other three, distortion also possible	100
Methyl isocyanide MeNC	Linear but with a very low electric field gradient at N, due presumably to a fortuitously favourable electronic structure	0.26
Methyl cyanide MeCN	Terminal	80
Pyridine C_5H_5N	Cyclic N	200
4-Methyl pyridine $CH_3C_5H_4N$	Molecular motion hindered by the substituent	480

Azide anion $:\overset{-}{N}=\overset{+}{N}=\overset{-}{N}:$	Central N	22
	Terminal N	55
^{17}O in:	$f(I, Q) = 0.000\ 22$	
The molybdate anion MoO_4^{2-}	Terminal but the electronic distribution gives an unexpectedly low field gradient	5
Ethanol EtOH	Typical of organic O	140
^{27}Al in:	$f(I, Q) = 0.007$	
The hexaaquoaluminium (III) cation $Al(H_2O)_6^{3+}$	Regular octahedron but with effects due to proton exchange	3 to 20
Aluminium *iso*-propoxide tetramer $[(Pr^iO)_2Al(\mu-OPr^i)_2]_3Al$	A central, octahedral Al connected to three, distorted tetrahedral Al via propoxide bridges	200 (octahedral) 3500 (tetrahedral)
Triisobutyl aluminium	Trigonal	6000
^{35}Cl in:	$f(I, Q) = 0.0083$	
Phosphorus trichloride PCl_3	Terminal atoms	83 000
The perchlorate anion ClO_4^-	Strictly regular tetrahedron	3
The chloride cation Cl^-	weakly interacting with water solvent	8

electro-asymmetry factors in the paramagnetic shielding term and the electric field gradient asymmetry are somehow related.

4.4.1   Spin—spin coupling to quadrupole relaxed nuclei

So far we have considered the effect that relaxation has upon line-width. Since T_1 relaxation involves changes in spin orientations we might also expect relaxation processes to modify the spin coupling patterns we observe. The relaxation times of spin $\frac{1}{2}$ nuclei are sufficiently long for us not normally to have to take this into account when analysing spectra, but the much shorter relaxation times of the quadrupolar nuclei do lead to considerable modification of the observed patterns.

If T_1 is long then the normal spin coupling effects are observed. Thus spin coupling of the methyl group to ^{11}B is observed in the adduct $MeNH_2BF_3$ though reference to Fig. 3.9 will show that the lines are rather broadened. At the other extreme, if T_1 is very short, the nuclear spins interchange energy and change orientation so rapidly, that a coupled nucleus interacts with all possible spin states in a short time. It can distinguish only an average value of the interaction and a singlet resonance results. This explains for instance why the chlorinated hydrocarbons show no evidence of proton spin coupling to the chlorine nuclei ^{35}Cl and ^{37}Cl, both with $I = 3/2$. At intermediate relaxation rates the coupling interaction is indeterminate and a broad line is observed. The line-shapes calculated for the resonance of a spin $\frac{1}{2}$ nucleus coupled to a quadrupole relaxed spin 1 nucleus such as ^{14}N are shown in Fig. 4.6. The shape of the spectrum observed depends upon the product T_1J, where T_1 is the relaxation time of the quadrupole nucleus, since if the frequency defined by $1/(2\pi T_1)$ is comparable with the coupling constant in Hz then the coupled nucleus cannot distinguish the separate spin states. The situation is equivalent to attempting to measure the frequency of a periodic wave by observing only a fraction of a cycle. The resonance of the quadrupolar nucleus will of course be split into a multiplet by the spin $\frac{1}{2}$ nuclei, but each component line will be broadened by its relaxation.

A common example of lines broadened by coupling to quadrupolar nuclei is found in amino compounds. The protons on the nitrogen are usually observed as a broad singlet, a good example appearing in Fig. 3.14b. It is important to remember in this case that the relaxation time of the amino proton is unaffected and can cause normal splitting in vicinal protons bonded to carbon. In contrast the protons in the

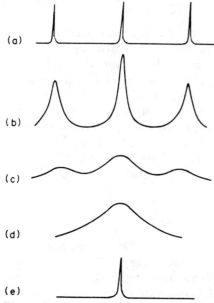

Figure 4.6   The resonance line-shape of a spin $\frac{1}{2}$ nucleus coupled to a spin 1 nucleus having various rates of quadrupole relaxation: (a) T_1 long; (b) $T_1 \approx 8/2\pi J$; (c) $T_1 \approx 3/2\pi J$; (d) $T_1 \approx 1/2\pi J$; (e) T_1 very short. The intensities are not to scale. The broadened lines are weak since the totals area is constant.

highly symmetrical ammonium ion give narrow resonances because the nitrogen quadrupole relaxation is slow (Fig. 3.7b).

Since quadrupole relaxation is sensitive to temperature and viscosity the line-shapes observed for coupled nuclei are altered by viscosity and temperature changes, an increase in temperature leading to *slower* relaxation and a better resolved multiplet. This fact is stressed since on a first encounter it appears to be contrary to one's expectation.

4.5   Other relaxation mechanisms

These are of importance for the spin $\frac{1}{2}$ nuclei with higher mass and low magnetic moments so that in the absence of ^{1}H or ^{19}F, dipole—dipole relaxation is virtually absent. Such nuclei, however, possess broadened resonances so that other relaxation mechanisms must intervene. These are summarized below, with the qualification that the number of proved examples of each type of process is relatively small.

4.5.1   *Spin rotation relaxation*

For small molecules which rotate rapidly or for rapidly rotating groups, a coupling exists between the nuclei and the molecular magnetic moment generated by the rotating charge distribution. Increased temperature increases the rate of rotation and the effective moment, and T_{1SR} decreases, in contrast to dipole–dipole relaxation where higher temperatures reduce the spectral density of the relaxation field. Thus a study of the temperature dependence of T_1 will enable the two mechanisms to be distinguished; often T_{1DD} predominates at low temperatures and T_{1SR} when the temperature is increased. This mechanism accounts for the broad resonances which are obtained from gaseous samples.

4.5.2   *Chemical shift anisotropy relaxation*

This has become important with the advent of the new very high field spectrometers. We have already discussed in Chapter 2 that the chemical shift of an atom depends upon the way the bonds to the atom interfere with the electronic circulation. Reference to Figs 2.2–2.5 will show that this depends upon the orientation of the molecule in the magnetic field and so is an anisotropic quantity. We observe a single value simply because the rapid tumbling of the molecule produces an average of all the possible screenings. In fact, because the nuclear screening changes as the molecule tumbles, there exists a small fluctuation in magnetic field at the nucleus which can cause relaxation. The mechanism is very inefficient but is proportional to $\mathbf{B}_0^2$. It thus produces a contribution for nuclei in a rather highly anisotropic environment and which possess large chemical shift ranges and then only at high fields. T_{1CSI} can be separated from other mechanisms by its magnetic field dependance. It leads to problems in carbon-13 spectroscopy with superconducting magnets, and in specific instances (e.g. $\sigma_\parallel - \sigma_\perp$ is ~7500 ppm for ^{199}Hg in Me_2Hg) at lower fields.

4.6   The spectrometer output, its detection and resonance line-shape

It is logical next to discuss the measurement of relaxation times. However we need first to know a little more of how the pulse spectrometer works and how relaxation affects the line-shape and width.

4.6.1 Relaxation processes following a 90° pulse

We have seen in Chapter 1 that a 90° pulse of the $\mathbf{B}_1$ field swings the precession cone axis out of the z direction into the xy plane, magnetization M_z becoming detectable magnetization M_{xy}. The spins now precess as a group in the xy plane at the Larmor frequency, but must relax to their original equilibrium position via the random relaxation field. This causes precession in all possible directions allowing the spins to both fan out in the xy plane so reducing M_{xy}, and to realign themselves around the z axis. In this way the spins spiral irregularly back to their precession cone around $\mathbf{B}_0$. Fortunately, we are not interested in the somewhat complex behaviour of individual spins but in the overall behaviour of M_z and M_{xy}.

Their return to equilibrium follows the exponential laws

$$(M_z)_t = (M_z)_\infty \left\{ 1 - \exp(-t/T_1) \right\} \tag{4.1}$$

i.e. M_z increases from zero to its equilibrium value, and

$$(M_{xy})_t = (M_{xy})_0 \exp(-t/T_2) \tag{4.2}$$

i.e. the transverse magnetization falls from its maximum value (equal to M_z) to zero after sufficient time has elapsed. This is summarized in Fig. 4.7. Immediately after the pulse, an output is obtained at the

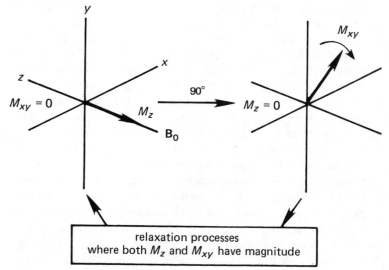

Figure 4.7 Perturbation of the spin orientation and relaxation to equilibrium.

nuclear frequency which diminishes in intensity but more rapidly than would be expected for the T_2 mechanism, since the inhomogeneities in the magnetic field within the sample due to magnet imperfections cause the spins to fan out even more rapidly. We write that the apparent relaxation time T_2^* is equal to

$$1/T_2^* = 1/T_2 + 1/T_{\text{inhomo}}$$

where the last term is the decay in intensity due to the inhomogeneities alone. Thus we cannot measure T_2 accurately from the rate of decay of the spectrometer output unless this is so short that the inhomogeneity contribution is negligible. T_1 is only manifested in changes which occur in intensity following a series of closely spaced pulses, too close to allow M_z to come to equilibrium. It will be evident that we need to design new experiments to measure T_1 and T_2.

We have already mentioned that the spectrometer output needs computer processing before it can be used. The nuclear frequency is too high for storage in a memory and we need to reduce this to the audio range. This is done using a phase sensitive detector.

4.6.2   The phase sensitive detector

This is a device which can be used to compare two periodic waves. The way it works is set out diagrammatically in Fig. 4.8. A change-over relay is driven by a square wave so that the output terminals are connected to the input in one sense during a positive half-cycle and in the opposite sense during the negative half-cycle. If a signal of the same frequency as the drive waveform is applied to the input this is rectified by the regular switching of the relay and a dc output is obtained if the two inputs are in phase or $180°$ out of phase. In the latter case the sign of the output is reversed. If the phase relationship of the two inputs is other than $0°$ or $180°$, an alternating component is obtained, but if this is integrated (or filtered) a dc output results but whose magnitude and sign depends upon the relative phases of the inputs. When the phase difference is $90°$ there is no dc output. If the input is the signal picked up from our nuclear magnets and the drive (or switching) wave form is obtained from the $\mathbf{B}_1$ drive oscillator, then an output is obtained which fluctuates from positive to negative at the difference frequency between that of the nuclear magnets and of $\mathbf{B}_1$ as these move in and out of phase, the faster vector continually passing the other. The output thus consists of an exponentially decaying waveform at a frequency low enough for computer processing. If the nuclei are exactly on resonance

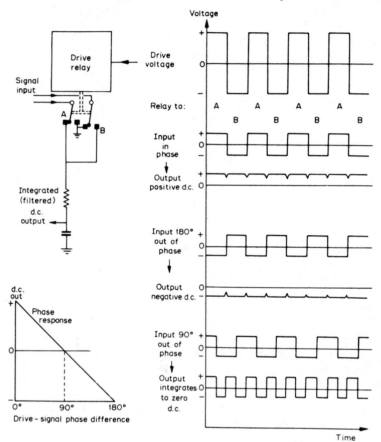

Figure 4.8   The phase sensitive detector. The output magnitude depends both upon the phase of the input relative to the drive and upon the magnitude of the input.

with the B_1 frequency, i.e. the nuclear vector and the B_1 vector have exactly the same angular velocity, then if they are in phase the output is not oscillatory but simply decays exponentially. If the two vectors are 90° out of phase, then there is no output. If the nuclear frequency and B_1 frequency are not the same then a decaying sinusoidal output is obtained whatever the phase relationship between the two, but of a phase depending on this relationship. This is summarized in Fig. 4.9.

In practice, electronic switching has to be used at nuclear frequencies and the drive waveform is used to make conducting alternatively first one and then the other pairs of diodes of a ring modulator so as to

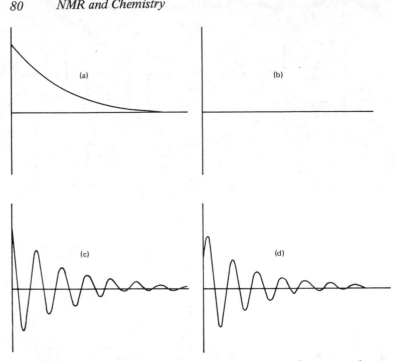

Figure 4.9   (a) and (b) illustrates the possible range of outputs when the nuclei are exactly on resonance with B_1 and are in phase (a) or $90°$ out of phase (b). If the nuclear and B_1 frequencies are different then the the output is at the difference frequency but starts on a maximum if they start in phase (c) or a minimum if they start $90°$ out of phase. Any intermediate phase is possible.

reverse the connection between a pair of transformers (Fig. 4.10). The output of course contains electronic noise as well as signal and this is minimized by the low pass filter which is constructed to allow the nuclear signals to pass (and the low frequency noise) but eliminates the predominant high frequency noise. A simple RC filter is included in Fig. 4.10.

4.6.3   Exponential relaxation and line-shape

The T_2 relaxation process means that the nuclear frequency is not precisely defined. The spins can be thought of as instantaneously having a frequency distribution around their resonance frequency ω_0 and a plot of this frequency distribution against frequency is the line shape $f(\omega)$ (Fig. 4.11). In fact the nuclei have quite random frequencies

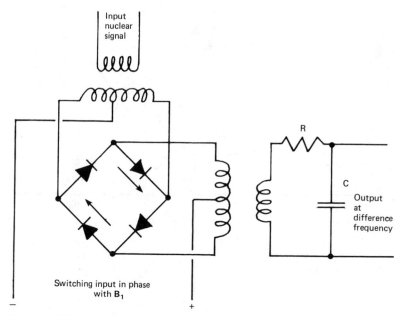

Figure 4.10   A typical phase sensitive detector circuit. With the switching input at the polarity shown, the two arrowed diodes conduct in the direction shown and connect the two transformers.

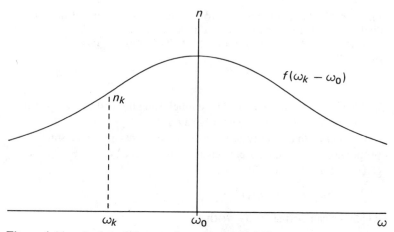

Figure 4.11   A plot of the number of nuclei with angular frequency ω_k different from the resonant frequency ω_0 for a small time interval t. The function $n_k = f(\omega_k - \omega_0)$ is the line-shape function.

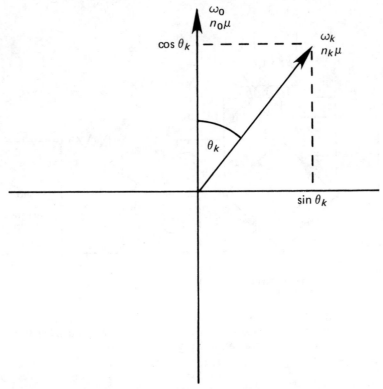

Figure 4.12   Showing how the total magnetic moment of the group of nuclei n_k with angular velocity ω_k is displaced an angle θ_k from the on resonance nuclei time t after a $\mathbf{B_1}$ pulse has produced magnetization in the xy plane.

within this range but over a short enough time interval we can picture them as having this quite regular behaviour.

If we have an assembly of N nuclei we can imagine that a small proportion n_k will have a particular angular velocity, ω_k. Each n_k is given by the line-shape function

$$n_k \propto f(\omega_k - \omega_0)$$

which we can normalize by writing

$$n_k = Nf(\omega_k - \omega_0) \tag{4.3}$$

i.e. we have chosen n_0 so that $\sum\limits_{k} f(\omega_k - \omega_0) = 1$.

At a small time t after the $\mathbf{B_1}$ pulse, those nuclei with angular velocity ω_k will have moved an angle θ_k from those nuclei exactly at resonance, ω_0 (Fig. 4.12). We can resolve the magnetic moments of the n_k nuclei along the ω_0 direction and at right angles to it, and following standard alternating current theory, we shall differentiate the normal component by the prefix i, where $i = \sqrt{-1}$.

We have that

$$\theta_k = (\omega_k - \omega_0)t$$

and the two components are

$$n_k \cos(\omega_k - \omega_0)t, \quad in_k \sin(\omega_k - \omega_0)t \tag{4.4}$$

The next step is to replace the n_k by the line-shape function. However, Fig. 4.9 indicates that these may not be the same for the two components and so we shall denote them as two separate functions by the letter letters v and u. The total intensity of the two components is then proportional to

$$Nv(\omega_k - \omega_0)\cos(\omega_k - \omega_0)t, \quad iNu(\omega_k - \omega_0)\sin(\omega_k - \omega_0)t \tag{4.5}$$

Summing over all possible values of k gives us the total intensity of each component. We normally would wish to compare this with the initial intensity at $t = 0$. This is proportional to the sum of all the nuclei, N. N thus cancels from the formulae. The intensity of the normal component is of course only significant if $\omega_0 \neq \omega_{\mathbf{B_1}}$. If N is large we can use the integral form of the equations which, remembering that ω is the variable, and t is constant, gives

$$\int_0^\infty v(\omega_k - \omega_0)\cos(\omega_k - \omega_0)t \, d\omega = e^{-t/T_2} \tag{4.6}$$

and

$$\int_0^\infty u(\omega_k - \omega_0)\sin(\omega_k - \omega_0)t \, d\omega = e^{-t/T_2} \tag{4.7}$$

It remains to find the form of the functions v and u. Inspection of tables of definite integrals will show that these are

$$u = \frac{(\omega_k - \omega_0)T_2^2}{1 + T_2^2(\omega_k - \omega_0)^2} \tag{4.8}$$

$$v = \frac{T_2}{1 + T_2^2(\omega_k - \omega_0)^2} \tag{4.9}$$

These two functions are plotted in Fig. 4.13. u is the dispersion and v is the absorption mode of the Lorenzian line-shape. The absorption signal has its maximum at ω_0 and its intensity is proportional to the number of nuclei producing the signal. The dispersion mode is of zero intensity at resonance and of different sign above and below resonance. Spectra are displayed in the absorption mode, though, as we shall see, the dispersion mode has an important use in spectrometer locking systems.

The problem remains of how to obtain the plots of Fig. 4.13 from the actual spectrometer output of Fig. 4.9. This is known as the free induction decay (FID) and is stored digitally in computer memory where it can easily be mathematically processed. Time and frequency domains are related through the Fourier relationship

$$F(\omega) = \int_{-\infty}^{\infty} f(t)e^{-i\omega t} dt \tag{4.10}$$

This can be written

$$F(\omega) = \int_{-\infty}^{\infty} f(t) \, (\cos \omega t - i \sin \omega t) dt \tag{4.11}$$

The Fourier transform of the output data thus contains two components, often called real and imaginery, which correspond to the u and v components. The inverse transform is also possible

$$f(t) = \frac{1}{2\pi} \int_{-\infty}^{\infty} F(\omega)e^{i\omega t} \, d\omega$$

and this should be compared with the relations 4.6 and 4.7 derived above.

4.6.4 Time and frequency domains

The output of an NMR spectrometer is a sinusoidal wave which decays with time. It varies entirely as a function of time and is said to exist in the time domain. Its initial intensity is proportional to M_z and so to the number of nuclei giving rise to the signal. Its frequency is a measure of its chemical shift and its rate of decay is related to T_2 and the quality of the magnetic field. Fourier transformation of this FID gives a function whose intensity varies as a function of frequency and is said to exist in the frequency domain. The parameters of the absorption curve contain all those of the FID: the position reproduces the frequency

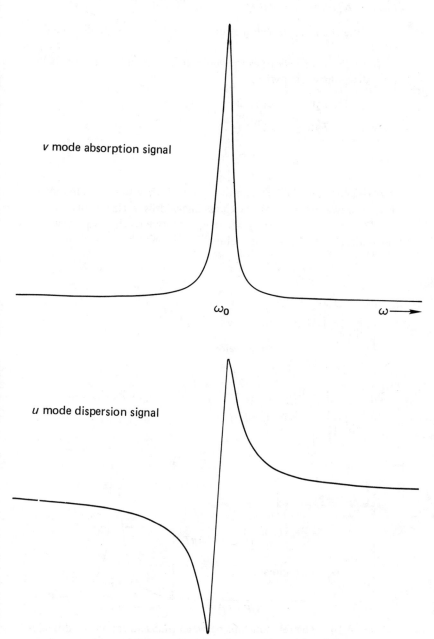

Figure 4.13   The absorption and dispersion mode signals available at the output of the phase sensitive detector (after transformation).

and so the chemical shift. Equation 4.9 can be used to predict the line-width.

If we define line-width as the width at half-intensity then the half-intensity points occur when:

$$1 + T_2^2(\omega_0 - \omega)^2 = 2$$

i.e. when $T_2^2(\omega_0 - \omega)^2 = 1$

or $$\omega_0 - \omega = \pm \frac{1}{T_2}$$

The separation of the half-intensity points is then twice this in radians. It is, however, more usual to express line-widths in Hz (frequency $= \omega/2\pi$) giving $\nu_{1/2} = 1/\pi T_2$ where $\nu_{1/2}$ represents the frequency separation of the half-height points. The line-width thus gives us $1/\pi T_2^*$.

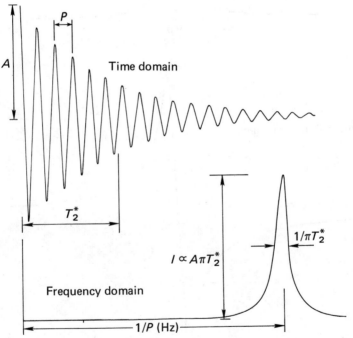

Figure 4.14   The relationships between time and frequency domains. The period P of the FID gives the position of the line. The rate of decay T_2^* gives the line-width and the initial amplitude A gives the line its area and therefore its intensity proportional to $A\pi T_2^*$.

The intensity of the absorption curve depends upon line-width, and in fact their product, or the area under the curve, are proportional to the initial FID intensity and so to the nuclear concentration. These relationships are summarized in Fig. 4.14.

4.7   Measurement of T_1 and T_2

Different experiments are required in order to measure T_1 and T_2, though if they are equal then measurement of T_1 suffices. However, in many systems of interest, T_2 is smaller than T_1 and we shall indicate how T_2 is measured also.

4.7.1   *Measurement of T_1 by population inversion*

This is the most popular of several available methods. We have already seen how a maximum NMR signal is obtained after a 90° $\mathbf{B_1}$ pulse. The same is obtained after a 270° pulse except that the spins have been inverted relative to the 90° pulse and the output is 180° out of phase with that after the shorter pulse. If we arrange our computer to give us a positive going absorption peak from the FID following a 90° pulse then after a 270° pulse we will get a negative peak. If instead, we use a 180° pulse, we create no M_{xy} but turn the excess low energy spins into the high energy state, $-M_z$. They will relax to their normal state with characteristic time T_1 and the magnetization will change from $-M_z$ through zero to $+M_z$ (Fig. 4.15). This of course produces no effects. However, if at some time τ (do not confuse this with τ_c) after the 180° pulse, we apply a second pulse of 90° we will create magnetization M_{xy} equal in magnitude to M_z at that instant. The spectrum that results from processing the FID will be negative going if M_z is still negative (as if part of the magnetization had undergone a 270° pulse) and positive going if M_z has passed through zero (Fig. 4.16). A series of spectra are obtained in this way for a number of different values of τ and the intensity of the resulting peaks plotted as a function of τ so allowing us to extract a value for T_1 (Fig. 4.17). Sufficient time must elapse between each 180/90° pair of pulses to allow M_z to relax fully to its equilibrium value or incorrect results will be obtained. Usually a waiting period of five to ten times T_1 is used. If T_1 is very long then the experiment can be very time consuming, but other pulse sequences have been worked out which will allow the total time to be reduced.

If there are several resonances in our spectrum, each relaxes at its own rate and it is possible with this method to measure the relaxation

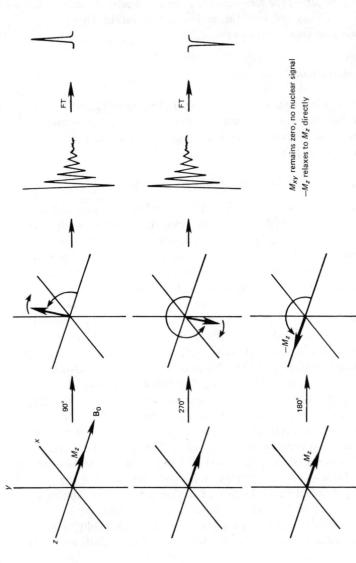

Figure 4.15   Upper: production of a nuclear response using a 90° pulse. Centre: a similar response is obtained after a 270° pulse but 180° out of phase giving an inverted transform. Lower: a 180° pulse gives no xy magnetization but places M_z in a non-equilibrium position opposing the field. This magnetization relaxes back to its equilibrium value and no transverse magnetization is produced at any time throughout the process.

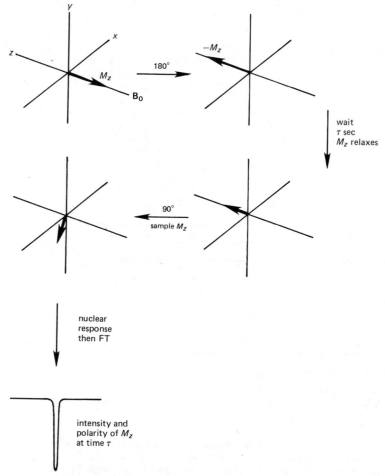

Figure 4.16   Showing how the pulse sequence $180° - $ wait $\tau - 90°$ can be used to perturb M_z and follow what then happens to M_z.

times of all the nuclei of the same isotope in a molecule and to obtain detailed information about molecular motion.

If the nuclei are spin coupled then the apparent relaxation times may not be simply related to the real ones. Carbon-13 relaxation times are commonly measured with the coupled protons 'decoupled' (discussed later) and this gives satisfactory results.

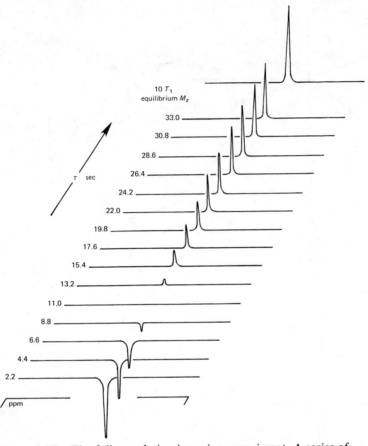

Figure 4.17   The full population inversion experiment. A series of spectra are obtained at different τ. A plot of their intensities as a function of time gives the rate of relaxation from which T_1 can be derived. (After Martin, Delpuech and Martin, *Practical NMR Spectroscopy*, John Wiley & Sons Inc., with permission.)

4.7.2   Measurement of T_2

The contribution of magnetic field inhomogeneity to T_2 will usually be of the order of 3.0 to 0.3 s for a high resolution magnet. Thus, provided T_2 is less than about 0.003 s it can be measured directly either from the line-width or from the rate of decay of the FID. In the last case we have to suppose that there is only a single resonance.

Accurate measurement of T_2 is made using a spin echo experiment.

It is required that $T_2 < T_1$. The spins fan out in the transverse plane due to two mechanisms, the random relaxation field and the fact that different parts of the sample experience different magnetic fields. This second is not a random process but continues predictably. We start by applying a 90° pulse and creating M_{xy}. The spins at different parts of the sample have different angular velocities and move away from the average, some going ahead and some lagging behind. We wait τ s and then apply a 180° pulse and tip the spins across to the other side of the xy plane. They move across as a bunch and continue to precess in their new position. However, now the slower ones are in front and the faster ones are behind so that they all move together again and reach a maximum M_{xy} at time 2τ after the 180° refocusing pulse. This process can be continued indefinitely and maxima in M_{xy} detected for as long as the random field relaxation allows M_{xy} to persist. The random processes cannot of course be refocused by such a technique. The intensity of the maxima or echoes thus falls at a rate determined by the real T_2. The spin behaviour is summarized in Fig. 4.18.

Each echo builds up in intensity to its maximum and then falls again so that the spectrometer output looks like a series of back to back FIDs. It is possible to separate each of these and Fourier transform it so that if the sample produces several resonances then the relaxation of each can be followed. Coupling must however be absent if the results are to be meaningful without having to resort to a full theoretical treatment of the system in question.

4.8   NMR spectra of dynamic systems

One of the most important contributions that NMR has made to chemistry is the insight it has given into the dynamic, time dependent nature of many systems, particularly those which are at equilibrium or where simply intramolecular motion is involved. Spectroscopy based on higher frequency radiation, such as classical IR or UV spectroscopy, has given mostly a static picture because the time-scale of many processes is slow relative to the frequency used. However, the lower frequencies used for NMR and the smaller line-separations involved, coupled with the small natural line-widths obtained, means that many time-dependent processes affect the spectra profoundly. We have of course already discussed one such process, namely quadrupole relaxation and how it affects spin coupling patterns.

If two atoms of the same element in a system have different chemical environments, then their nuclei (assuming these are the same species)

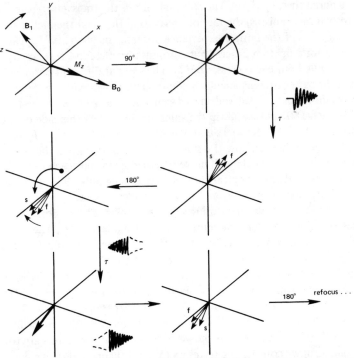

Figure 4.18   Illustrating the Carr-Purcell pulse sequence for measuring T_2. The behaviour of the spins is shown relative to $\mathbf{B}_1$, as if they were stationary. The 90° pulse produces M_{xy} which then decreases as the spins move apart, s = slow, f = fast. The 180° pulse alters the position of the slower and faster spins which now close up again and M_{xy} increases and then decreases.

will give rise to two chemically shifted resonance lines. If the atoms interchange position occasionally, their lifetime τ in any one environment is long and the spectrum is hardly altered. On the other hand if the lifetime is exceptionally short then the spectrometer can only distinguish an average environment and a singlet is observed. At intermediate lifetimes a broadened line is obtained whose shape is determined by $\tau \nu_0 \delta$, where δ is the ppm chemical shift between the resonances in the absence of exchange.

An example of this behaviour is found with the N-methyl resonance of N,N-dimethylformamide, $Me_2 N.CHO$. This is a doublet at 25° because rotation around the C—N bond is restricted since the nitrogen lone pair electrons form a partial double bond to the carbonyl carbon, and the two methyl groups lie in different chemical environments (Fig. 4.19). If the compound is heated the rate of rotation increases and

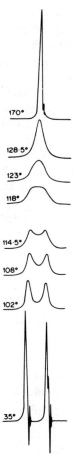

Figure 4.19 The N-methyl resonance of N, N-dimethyl-formamide
neat liquid at different temperatures. Rotation of the Me_2N groups
around the CN bond is slow at room temperature due to partial double-
bond character in the bond.

At high temperatures the barrier to rotation is overcome and the two
methyl groups see the same average environment. The spectrum at $118°$
where the doublet structure is just lost is said to be at coalescence.
(Reproduced with permission from Bovey (1965) *Chem. and Eng.
News*, Aug. 30, 103.)

the line-shapes change in the way shown in the figure. It is possible to observe these changes, albeit somewhat crudely, if a heated sample is placed in the coil of certain NMR spectrometers and a series of spectra obtained rapidly as the sample cools.

Line-widths and spectral shapes change quite profoundly with temperature, and for this reason considerable effort has been put into the determination of exchange rates from spectral shapes, so that activation parameters can be obtained from Arrhenius type temperature—rate plots. In order to do this of course a quantitative theory of the method is required. We do not intend to discuss this here but simply to give certain particular results relating to certain situations. If exchange is slow and if we consider exchange between two sites A and B where the residence times on each site are τ_A and τ_B and the relaxation times are T_{2A} and T_{2B}, respectively, then the apparent relaxation time T_2' is reduced as follows at each site

$$\frac{1}{T_{2A}'} = \frac{1}{T_{2A}} + \frac{1}{\tau_A}$$

$$\frac{1}{T_{2B}'} = \frac{1}{T_{2B}} + \frac{1}{\tau_B}$$

(4.12)

i.e. two broadened lines are obtained. The broadening arises because the leaving spin does not necessarily have the same orientation as the arriving spin so that extra relaxation is introduced.

For fast exchange we define the proportions of A and B sites as P_A and P_B where:

$$P_A = \frac{\tau_A}{\tau_A + \tau_B} \qquad P_B = \frac{\tau_B}{\tau_A + \tau_B}$$

(4.13)

then

$$\frac{1}{T_2'} = \frac{P_A}{T_{2A}} + \frac{P_B}{T_{2B}} + P_A^2 P_B^2 (2\pi\nu_0\delta)^2 (\tau_A + \tau_B)$$

(4.14)

giving a single broadened line of resonant frequency:

$$\nu' = P_A \nu_A + P_B \nu_B$$

at the weight averaged shift position. These two expressions can be used to gain a rough idea of exchange rates in the two limiting cases though magnetic field inhomogeneities make the results very inaccurate.

These equations do not apply in the region of spectral collapse where the factors involved are more complex ($108° - 123°$ in Fig. 4.19).

It should be noted how clearly defined, in terms of temperature, is the coalescence point, the point where multiplet structure is just lost, to within $\pm 2°$ or so. We have at coalescence, the coalescence residence time τ_c

$$\tau_c = \frac{\sqrt{2}}{\pi(\nu_0\delta)}, \text{ where } 2/\tau_c = 1/\tau_A + 1/\tau_B,$$

and this gives us a very precise relationship between temperature and exchange rate since we avoid the errors inherent in measuring line-widths when we apply Equations 4.12 or 4.14. The existence today of multinuclear spectrometers and spectrometers operating at different magnetic fields allows us to measure τ_c for several values of $\nu_0\delta$ and so obtain data with maximum accuracy. An example using two resonances from a molecule, ^1H and ^{13}C spectroscopy to give an Arrhenius plot with eight points is illustrated in Fig. 4.20 for $Et_2NCS_2Fe(CO)_2(C_5H_5)$.

The ^1H spectra consist of two ethyl (triplet–quartet) patterns since the ethyl group *trans* to SFe is in a different environment to the one *cis*. Exchange by rotation around the C—N bond merges the two

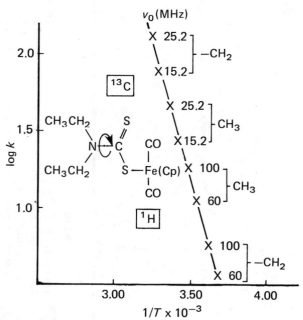

Figure 4.20   Determination of the activation parameters characterizing the hindered rotation around the C—N bond of $(CH_3CH_2)_2N$—CS—S—$Fe(CO)_2$ Cp (Cp = cyclopentadienyl).

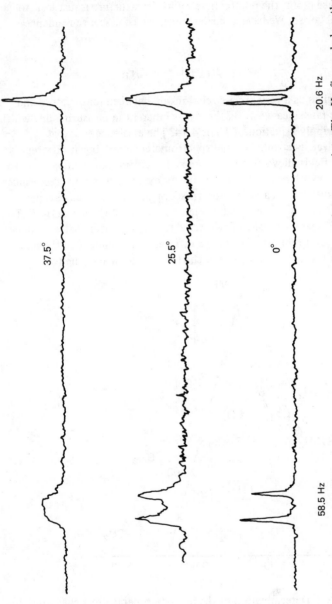

58.5 Hz

20.6 Hz

Figure 4.20 (*continued*) ^{13}C spectra at 25.2 MHz illustrating two of the coalescence points. The Hz figures below the traces give the line separations in the slow exchange limit. The methyl carbon resonance is on the right, the methylene on the left. All other resonances are omitted for clarity. (Graph reproduced with permission from Martin, Delpuech and Martin *Practical NMR Spectroscopy*, p. 342 and spectra supplied by the Authors.).

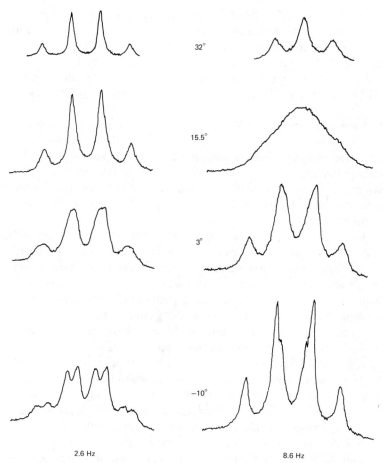

32°

15.5°

3°

−10°

2.6 Hz

8.6 Hz

Figure 4.20 (*continued*) The coalescences in the 100 MHz proton spectra. The methylene resonances are on the left and methyl on the right. Note that at low temperatures the two triplets of the latter overlap and two of the lines appear as shoulders on the intense central lines.

patterns into a single ethyl pattern. The chemical shift between the two methyl or two methylene multiplets are different so that their coalescence temperatures are different and we obtain two points on the Arrhenius plot. The chemical shifts in Hz also change with magnetic field and we can obtain four points by using spectrometers working at 100 MHz and 60 MHz. The carbon spectra are obtained as singlets by

decoupling the protons (see Chapter 7) and are much more widely
separated than the proton resonances and so give four more points with
the same spectrometers, at higher temperatures. The Arrhenius
equation $\ln k = \ln A - E_a/RT$ leads to the values $E_a = 66$ kJ mole^{-1}
and $\ln A = 13.1$ whence we can calculate $\Delta H^* = 63.8$ kJ mole^{-1} and
$\Delta S^* = -2.3$ J mole^{-1} deg^{-1}. The rate constants are obtained from
$k = 1/\tau_c$.

Variable temperature NMR spectroscopy has been used extensively
to study many dynamic processes. The rates of exchange involved and
line-separations vary considerably, so that some samples require cooling
rather than heating to reach the temperature where the exchange rate
affects the form of the NMR spectra. Because of the importance of this
type of work many spectrometers are equipped with devices for cooling
or heating the sample.

In such spectrometers the sample is placed in a Dewar-jacketed probe
and heated or cooled nitrogen gas passed through the probe. Typically,
temperatures in the range $+ 200°$C to $- 130°$C can be achieved though
temperature control is never so good as in a conventional thermostatic
bath, due mainly to the low thermal capacity of the heat exchange
medium. For the same reason one cannot guarantee that the whole of
the sample is at the same temperature. Despite these drawbacks, much
interesting information about exchange processes has emerged using
variable temperature NMR spectroscopy. Studies have for instance been
made of the hindered rotation which occurs around the carbon—carbon
bond in highly halogenated ethanes, of the flexing of saturated rings
and of the exchange of ligands on transition metal complexes. Several
further examples will be described in detail in Chapter 9.

NMR can also be used to study protolysis reactions. In a pure
alcohol, RCH_2OH, the methylene protons are coupled both to protons
in R and to the OH group. Thus in the spectrum of pure ethanol
(Fig. 4.21a) the hydroxyl and CH_2 resonances are broadened due to
this coupling. The coupling is not fully resolved except in very pure
samples because of slow interchange of hydroxide protons. Addition of
a drop of hydrochloric acid promotes faster exchange and the loss of
all coupling interaction since the hydroxide protons are replaced
frequently with random spin orientation. The resulting dramatic line-
narrowing is seen in Fig. 4.21b. The exchange rates of the protons in
such systems have been studied as a function of acid concentration by
analysing the line-shapes obtained.

The spectra of ethanol also illustrate the effects upon NMR spectra
of chemical equilibria involving fast exchange. The hydroxy group of

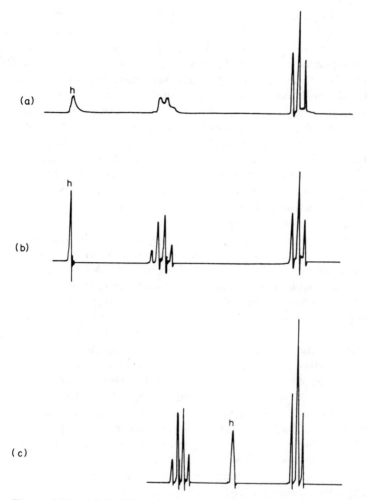

Figure 4.21   (a) 60 MHz proton spectrum of neat ethanol. The methyl
protons give rise to the triplet at high field and the methylene protons
give the quartet near the centre of the spectrum. Hydroxyl exchange is
slow and the methylene quartet is broadened by partially collapsed spin
coupling to the hydroxyl proton. This likewise gives a broadened singlet
at low field labelled h. (b) A drop of hydrochloric acid markedly
increases the rate of hydroxyl proton exchange and all vestiges of
coupling between hydroxyl and methylene protons are destroyed. The
hydroxyl (h) and methylene resonances sharpen dramatically. (c) A
dilute (~ 7%) solution of ethanol in deutero chloroform. The solvent
breaks up the intermolecular hydrogen bonds that exist in the neat
liquid and the hydroxyl resonance (h) moves 2.8 ppm upfield.

the alcohol is extensively inter-molecularly hydrogen-bonded. The degree of hydrogen bonding is not however 100%, so that the hydroxyl protons can be thought of simply as existing in two environments, one hydrogen-bonded and one non-hydrogen-bonded. Two resonances might be observed but for the fact that there is rapid interchange of hydroxyl roles, and a single line is observed at a position determined by the concentration-weighted average of the shifts in the two environments. If the degree of hydrogen bonding is altered then the resonance should move. A change in hydrogen bonding is brought about by diluting the alcohol in an organic solvent and a large hydroxyl shift is observed in Fig. 4.21c. The more extensively hydrogen-bonded neat alcohol has the lower field hydroxyl resonance (the methyl and methylene resonances are affected relatively little). Hydrogen bonding results in a low field shift possibly because of an electric field effect.

The hydrated proton resonates at very low field, and the addition of acid to water results in fast proton exchange between solvent and hydrated proton and a low field shift of the water resonance. This phenomenon has been used to study the dissociation of strong acids.

The destruction of spin coupling by exchange requires a further word. In the example given, the exchange involved bond breaking and replacement of one proton by another of not necessarily the same spin orientation. Thus the exchange can be regarded as leading to apparent nuclear relaxation. Exchange not involving bond rupture can however also affect spin coupling. If the coupling constant between two nuclei in a molecule is different for two conformations of the molecule, then if conformational interchange occurs the coupling will not be destroyed. If the exchange is slow, two molecular species will be present and two multiplet sets will be seen, one corresponding to each conformation. If exchange is fast then the corresponding lines of each multiplet set will be averaged and a single multiplet set will be obtained exhibiting average coupling constants and an average shift.

An important example of this is the spectrum of the ethyl grouping. The six vicinal coupling constants existing at any instant between the three methyl protons and the two methylene protons will be different since all the dihedral angles will be different; the chemical shifts of all the protons may also be different and a complex spectrum should result. Rapid rotation of the methyl groups however averages all the different couplings over a Karplus curve and also averages the shifts, so that only one coupling constant is observed. The three methyl protons are all magnetically equivalent and so are the two methylene protons. In considering equivalence of nuclei such rapid molecular motion should always be taken into account.

An important exception where rotation cannot lead to complete averaging is found for methylene protons which are bound to a carbon atom which is bonded to another carbon atom carrying three different substituents, i.e. $RCH_2-CR_1R_2R_3$. The presence of the substituent R on the methylene carbon means that the methylene protons are never in exactly the same environment whatever the conformation and an AB spectrum results. Note that the methylene protons may remain inequivalent if R_1 is a second CH_2R group. Thus the presence of an asymmetric carbon is not essential for this type of inequivalence to occur.

Slow chemical reactions where the reactants are not in equilibrium, in contrast to the above cases, can of course also be followed using NMR, though in this case a series of normal spectra are obtained over a period of time with no evident exchange perturbation, except that the relative line intensities vary and some lines may disappear and new ones appear. Reactions taking upwards of 60 s can be studied in this way.

More recently, some workers have adapted stopped flow devices to NMR spectroscopy. The two reacting solutions are held in reservoirs in the magnetic field so as to allow the nuclei to polarize and develop M_z. They are then mixed in the NMR tube within a few milliseconds and a series of spectra run and the FIDs stored sequentially in computer memory for later transformation into spectra. Reactions which are complete in about 5 s can be studied by stopped flow and examples are on record using the nuclei ^1H and ^{27}Al.

5
Modern Spectrometer Systems

We have already outlined at the end of Chapter 1 how a Fourier transform spectrometer works and have indicated that magnetic field homogeneity and stability must be of the highest standard. We shall take these as being satisfactory here though we will have to return to the problem of field stability again when we have discussed fully the various spectrometer systems. We have also shown how the phase sensitive detector works in Chapter 4, and why it is used, and this will not be mentioned further in this chapter.

5.1 Time and frequency domains

We have already encountered in Chapter 4 the concept of time and frequency domains and how the form of the FID is related to the transformed resonance line (Fig. 4.14). We will expand on this theme here to enable us to better understand the features of more complex spectra.

Thus a single cosine wave, $v = a \cos \omega t$ is represented in the frequency domain by a single frequency, ω (Fig. 5.1a). If we modulate the amplitude of this wave by a periodic wave of lower frequency, ϕ, such that the amplitude varies from 0 to $2a$, then we have $v = a(1 + \cos \phi t) \cos \omega t$, which on expansion gives:

$$v = \tfrac{1}{2}a \cos \omega t + \tfrac{1}{4}a \cos(\omega - \phi)t + \tfrac{1}{4}a \cos(\omega + \phi)t$$

so that the modulation has produced two new frequencies in the frequency representation of the wave, Fig. 5.1b. This simple example serves to illustrate that (a) an infinite wave is represented by a single pure frequency (the precision which we can define the frequency depends on how long we are willing to spend in its measurement) and (b) that distortion of the wave in the time domain results in the production of extra frequencies around the original carrier wave frequency, called side bands. This is a general phenomenon, and one way of stating the Fourier theorem is to say that any periodic function of time, however complex, may be synthesized from a suitable combination of pure cosine waves. In other words, it has a frequency spectrum. If the function of time only persists for a limited time, then this limits the precision with which its frequency may be known and the spectral components have width and intensity which may exist over a very wide frequency range. The Lorenzian transform of an FID is a case in point (Fig. 4.14). Modulation of an FID, or interference, indicates that it contains several well defined frequencies and some simple patterns are indicated in Fig. 5.1 for sets of equally spaced frequencies. We note that the sextet pattern begins to resemble a train of pulses and are not surprised to find that a series of well spaced, narrow rectangular pulses, such as is used to generate a series of FID responses, consists of an infinite series of frequencies separated by the inverse of the time between pulses. The separation is infinitely small for a single isolated pulse and the spectrum is then continuous with the same bandshape whose width is inversely proportional to the pulsewidth. So we see how the short pulses used in NMR spectroscopy spread the available radio frequency energy over a very large bandwidth and why all the chemically shifted nuclei in a sample are subject to the same B_1 field at their own frequency and all precess equally around B_1. Only if the chemical shift range is very large, or the pulsewidth is long is the B_1 field likely to be different at different nuclei. Practical pulselengths are usually less than 100 μs so that B_1 is of high amplitude over at least 10 000 Hz and we need only worry about the precise bandshape if we require quantitive data. We also see that since all the nuclei respond simultaneously, the response in the time domain will be complex and that a computer analysis will be needed in order to sort out all the component frequencies.

5.2   The collection of data in the time domain

In order to carry out numerical processing of the output of an NMR spectrometer we need to convert the analogue electrical output into digital information using an analogue—digital converter (A/D converter).

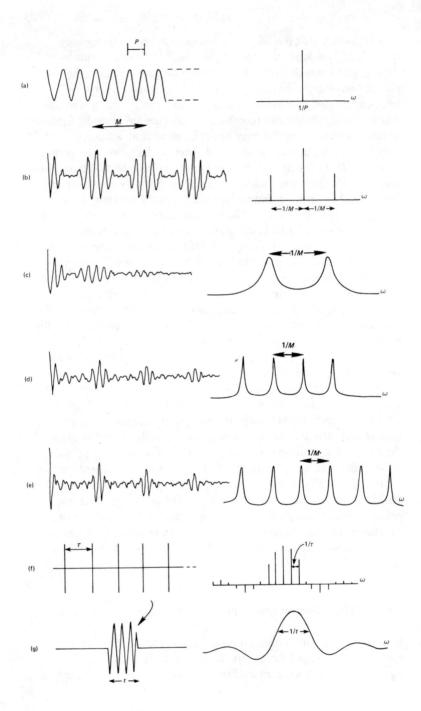

The signal is sampled at regular intervals, the voltage registered converted into a binary number, and this number then stored sequentially in one of a series of computer memory locations, one location being a word of 16 or 20 bits (Fig. 5.2). The magnitude of the sampling interval is very important, and is often known as the dwell time, DW. The maximum frequency that sampled information can represent is limited to that where alternate numbers are positive and negative — assuming a cosine wave input varying symmetrically about zero. The period of this wave is then $2(DW)$ and its frequency is $1/[2(DW)] = F$. A lower frequency, $F - f$, or a higher frequency, $F + f$, gives the same pattern in memory so that there is an ambiguity in the digital representation of the signals. This is avoided by ensuring that all the nuclear frequencies lie in the range 0 to F Hz. This is often known as the sweep width or as the spectral width. F is known generally as the Nyquist frequency.

Given that the spectrometer is highly stable, a series of isolated 90° pulses will each give an identical nuclear response so that these can be

---

Figure 5.1   The relationship between some time domain signals (on the left) and their Fourier transforms. (a) A continuous cosine wave of period P gives a single infinitely narrow line at frequency $1/P$. (b) If a cosine wave of period P is intensity modulated by a second wave of period M the line at frequency $1/P$ is flanked by two lines of half the intensity and separated from the centreband by $\pm 1/M$ Hz. (c) If the intensity of the wave decays rapidly to zero, the lines then have width. Two components give a modulated, decaying pattern with the separation between maxima now being M and the separation between the lines $1/M$. (d) and (e) The same relationship holds for groups of equally spaced lines of equal intensity. Note however, that the energy in the wave pattern becomes more and more concentrated at the maxima as the number of lines is increased, and begins to resemble a train of pulses. (f) A train of rectangular pulses like that of example (g) then has a multiple line transform though if the train does not diminish in intensity with time then the lines are infinitely narrow. They are separated by $1/\tau$ Hz, where τ is the pulse spacing but have a curious distribution because the pulses are rectangular. The intensities follow a sinc curve, where $\mathrm{sinc}X = (\sin X)/X$, and some have negative values. This means that they are 180° out of phase with the positive intensities. The width of the central band, where the intensity is greatest, is $1/t$ Hz, where t is the length of the rectangular pulse. We thus see that a train of rectangular pulses provides a band of B_1 frequencies which can be used to perturb all the chemically shifted nuclei in a sample. (g) A single rectangular pulse has infinite τ so that the frequencies fuse to form a continuum following the sinc curve with width $1/t$ at the centre band.

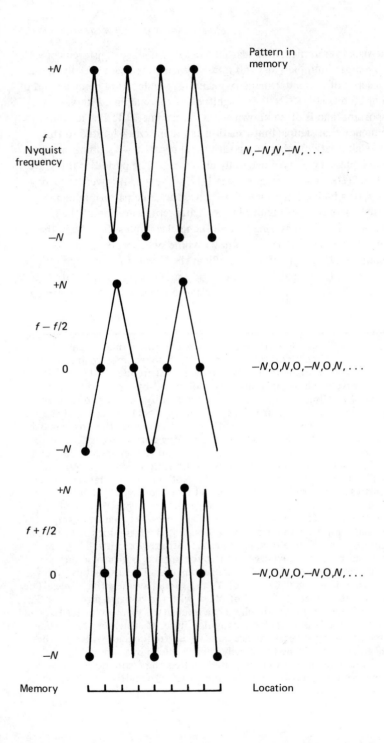

Pattern in memory

+N

f
Nyquist
frequency

$N, -N, N, -N, \ldots$

−N

+N

f − f/2

0

$-N, O, N, O, -N, O, N, \ldots$

−N

+N

f + f/2

0

$-N, O, N, O, -N, O, N, \ldots$

−N

Memory

Location

added together in the computer memory to give a much stronger total response. Each signal is, however, accompanied by unwanted random noise, indeed weak signals may not be visible because of the noise, and while the noise intensity also increases as more responses are added, the noise is incoherent, i.e. its intensity at a given memory location is sometimes + and sometimes −, then it adds up relatively slowly. A series of N FIDs when added together in this way has a signal to noise ratio which is $\sqrt{N}$ times better than that of a single FID. It is this feature which renders Fourier transform spectroscopy so useful for the less receptive nuclei, allowing a response to be collected from an apparently hopeless morass of noise. Fig. 5.3.

5.2.1   Memory size

The time during which a single FID may be collected is limited by the finite size of the computer memory. If there are M locations then they will all have been traversed after $M(DW)$ seconds. Since, strictly, we should wait until $5T_1$ seconds have elapsed before we apply the next pulse, we may also have to introduce a waiting time. Thus a standard FT experiment can be summarized by Fig. 5.4. The size of the memory does not affect the spectral width. After transformation of the accumulated FID, the dispersion and absorption parts of the spectrum each occupy $M/2$ locations of the same memory (this gives maximum utilization of expensive memory space) and the smallest frequency interval which can be detected is $2F/M$ Hz. Memory size therefore determines the resolution. If lines are closer than $2F/M$ they can never be separated. We note that $2F/M$ is equal to $1/M(DW)$, the time for which we observe an individual response, and that it is a fundamental fact that if we observe a response for only t seconds then our resolution cannot be better than $1/t$ Hz. Any line narrower than this limit will be represented by a single point in the transform and its absorption intensity may be zero if its frequency falls between two locations, though the broad wings of the dispersion part will still be visible.

Figure 5.2   Upper: showing how a waveform at the Nyquist frequency, f, gives alternate positive and negative values of the number N corresponding to peak voltage. This assumes that the wave and the computer memory sweep are in a certain timing relationship. Centre: a waveform of lower frequency, $f - f/2$, gives a different pattern. Lower: a waveform higher than the Nyquist frequency and by the same amount, $f + f/2$, gives exactly the same pattern.

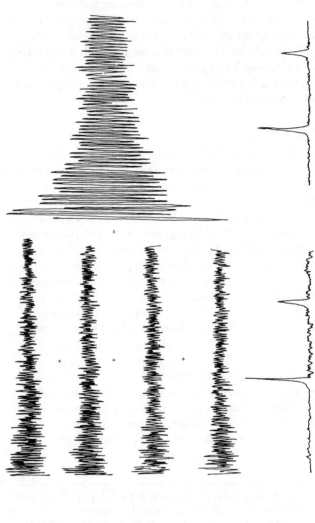

Figure 5.3   Four separate FIDs were collected and stored in memory, and these are plotted at the top left of the figure. The FID becomes indistinguishable from noise about one third the way along and has only twice the noise intensity even right at the start. The sum of the four FIDs is shown at the top right and the signal now starts with an intensity which is much larger than noise. The Fourier transforms of the sum and of a single initial FID are shown below. The theoretical improvement for four FIDs is two times, though in this particular example, some large noise fluctuations seem to have been fortuitously suppressed.

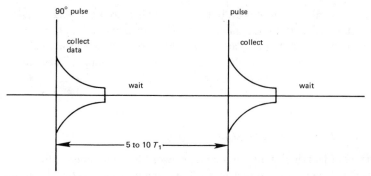

Figure 5.4 The ideal FT experiment which allows the spins to relax to equilibrium before successive pulses are applied. The data are collected until the memory is completely traversed.

Adequate resolution is therefore essential for full definition of the spectrum — each line must be represented by several points.

5.2.2 Rapid multiple pulsing

The waiting time needed to allow the spin system to come to equilibrium is a waste of our equipment since it is quiescent while waiting. It was quickly found that the signal to noise ratio can be maximized in a given time if we adopt the procedure:

pulse — acquire data — pulse — acquire . . .

with no waiting time at all; i.e. we allow the computer acquisition time to determine the pulse repetition rate. If this time is shorter than T_1, as is often the case for spin $\frac{1}{2}$ nuclei, we find that some magnetization M_{xy} exists when the successive pulses after the first are applied. If these are 90° pulses then the later ones will tip the magnetization through the xy plane and so reduce the signal intensity. The signal strength is then optimized by reducing the length of the pulse until a maximum 'steady state' output is achieved (i.e. the initial FID intensities are steady and as large as possible). The pulse lengths commonly found practicable are in the range 45° to 30°, depending on nucleus, chemical shift range, T_1 and memory size. However, the relaxation times of chemically shifted nuclei are often quite different so that the optimum pulselength will be different for each and the intensity of each type of resonance will depend upon its T_1. Thus if accurate quantitive data is required the ideal sequence depicted in Fig. 5.4 will have to be used. Happily, this is not too stringent a limitation in many cases since we know that a given molecule will contain integral numbers of atoms, but it does have to be born in mind and a particular experiment carried out with the final objectives in view. We should also note that rapid pulsing disturbs spin populations and can distort the shapes of spin–spin multiplets.

5.2.3   Dynamic range and word length

The word length of a binary number or word is the number of binary bits which can make up that word. Two such parameters concern us in FT spectroscopy; the word length of the memory and the word length that the A/D converter provides for the maximum input that it can handle.

If the digitizer has a word length of, say, 9 bits and the memory one of 20 bits, then if the input activates all the bits of the digitizer we can collect a maximum of $2^{11} = 2048$ FIDs. If we wish to improve the noise level more than such a number permits ($32\sqrt{2}$ times) then we have to reduce the amplitude of the input. If the signal is not visible in the noise it is sufficient that the noise activates only the first bits of the digitizer. The presence of the coherent signal will then ensure that on average the output number is positive more often than negative when the signal is positive so that eventually the signal will emerge, though this is limited by the size of the memory word (which limits the number of accumulations which can be carried out in the absence of special techniques which we will not discuss here). The digitizer word length also determines the minimum voltage that it can detect, that voltage which will just activate the least significant bit. Any signal weaker than this limit will not be detectable. Thus a weak signal will not be detectable if it is below a certain level relative to a strong one since this limits the extent to which we can increase the input to the A/D converter. We say that the dynamic range is limited by the A/D converter word length, and this is made as large as possible, commonly 12 bits. In addition, because the memory word size may limit the number of scans possible in the presence of a strong signal, the ability to observe a weak signal may be even further limited.

Now, the reason for the high sensitivity of the FT spectrometer, and therefore its success with the less receptive nuclei, is the fact that it sees all the nuclear responses simultaneously and does not take any time in searching the frequency domain for them. The method is thus ideal for biological samples where it is required to investigate the weak responses from large and complex molecules. Unfortunately, such molecules have to be studied in aqueous media and while the water signal strength is minimized by using D_2O as solvent, there are sufficient exchangeable protons in such samples to give rise to a strong proton signal, and so reduce the dynamic range that we can investigate. One way to improve matters is to design our experiment on the pulse sequence devised to measure T_1, namely $180° - \tau - 90° -$ collect. Here we take advantage of the fact that the T_1 of water and of our molecule will be different. We adjust τ so that the water spin magnetization is just zero at the time of the $90°$ pulse and so lose the water signal. The other signals accumulate in memory in the usual way except that their signal intensity is reduced because their magnetization will not have recovered to its equilibrium value by the time of the $90°$ pulse.

This disadvantage is overcome by using some form of selective pulse. If we use a weak $\mathbf{B_1}$ pulse, which can therefore be of very long duration, then this covers a very small frequency range — a pulselength of 1 s has a width of 1 Hz for instance — and can be tuned to a given resonance in the spectrum. We then tune this frequency to the water resonance, apply a $180°$ pulse which will tip only the water protons, wait till the water magnetization is zero and then apply the normal strong, non-selective pulse and collect data containing a minimum contribution from the solvent (Fig. 5.5). The intensity is then only reduced in the region close to the water resonance.

5.2.4 *Manipulation of the collected data*

FT NMR involves the collection of data in a computer memory. Now a computer is an infinitely variable instrument; it will do anything that you wish to the data that it contains, provided that you possess a suitable program. The minicomputers used for NMR spectroscopy have a section of memory containing programs as well as memory used simply for data accumulation, and many have in addition a backing store in the form of a disk or magnetic tape. Thus a set of data which may have taken several hours to acquire can be stored in permanent form and recalled to allow a variety of methematical processes to be carried out with the object of improving the data in a variety of ways. Indeed, the most up to date computers now allow foreground—background working where data may be accumulated by part of the memory while previously obtained data is being processed in another part.

The most commonly used technique is to multiply the data by an

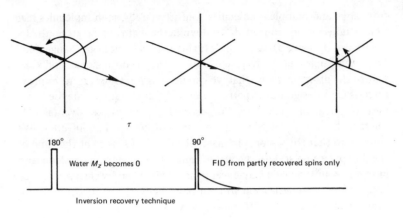

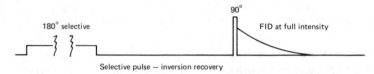

Figure 5.5   Means of eliminating a strong solvent response in the FT experiment. Inversion recovery: a non-selective 180° pulse turns all the spins against B_0, solvent (full vector) and solute (dotted vector) together. After time τ when the solvent M_z has become zero, a 90° pulse tips the solute vector, which has relaxed more rapidly, into the xy plane and a signal is obtained. The selective pulse does not affect the solute, only the solvent, and the full response to the 90° pulse is obtained.

exponentially decaying function, $k = e^{-n/K}$, where the multiplying factor k to use on the number stored in memory location n decreases from unity as the function moves along the data, starting from the point where data collection commences. The constant K is a pseudo time constant related to the size of the data treated and the rate at which it is desired to decrease the intensity of the data. The process is illustrated in Fig. 5.6. This treatment increases the rate of decay of the FID and so broadens the lines obtained after Fourier transformation. This disadvantage is acceptable, however, because the signal to noise ratio is also improved. We can see that this arises qualitatively since in the early part of the FID the signal is much larger than the noise and this part of the data is little affected by the multiplication; the signal may however be hardly visible in the tail of the FID and here the multiplication reduces markedly the importance of this part. The effect

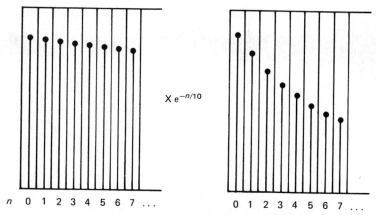

$X e^{-n/10}$

Figure 5.6 Illustrating the way exponential multiplication is carried out in a computer. The boxes represent memory locations where numbers are stored, represented by the sticks. The slowly decaying function on the left is multiplied successively by $e^{-0.1}$, $e^{-0.2}$, $e^{-0.3}$, ... for $n = 1, 2, 3, \ldots$ to give a more rapidly decaying function. Data collection is started in location 0, and n and time increase together after the pulse.

of the process is illustrated in Fig. 5.7. It allows the signal to noise ratio to be increased in a time that is very much shorter than required to accumulate extra data, provided that the loss in resolution is not important.

The Fourier transform of the exponentially decaying function is a Lorenzian line and we can also regard the line broadening as arising from a mixing of this with the spectral lines in the frequency domain. Such a mixing process is called convolution and in this case convolution is carried out by multiplying the spectrum by a Lorenzian function and storing the result, then moving the function along one place in the memory and repeating the multiplication and storing the new result, etc. (Fig. 5.8). This gives exactly the same result as exponential multiplication but is rather more time consuming so is seldom used. Convolution with a simple square function is, however, a means of cleaning up the noise which can be used after Fourier transformation if this should prove necessary and can avoid having to reprocess all the data again.

Where the FID is rather short lived (T_2 small) it is often best to use a short dwell time so as to spread the data out in memory. This means that the first data point is collected very shortly after the end of the B_1 pulse, and, due to the imperfections of electronic circuitry, there is

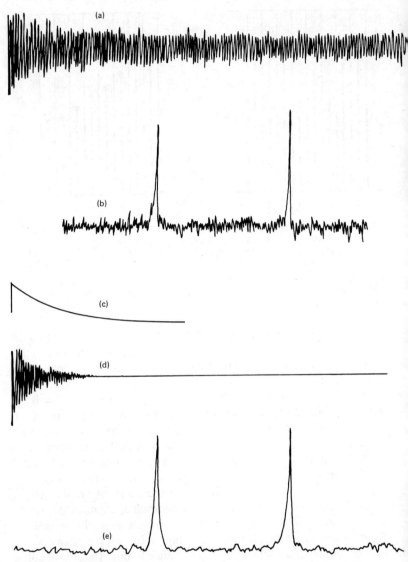

Figure 5.7 The effect of the exponential process. (a) A noisy FID where the signal quickly disappears below the noise and (b) its transform. This FID is multiplied by the falling exponential (c) to give (d) where the most noisy part of the FID is much reduced, as is the noise in the transform (e) which is about half the intensity of that in (b) and smoothed. The decay rate of (c) was chosen to approximate that in the signal and is known then as a matched filter.

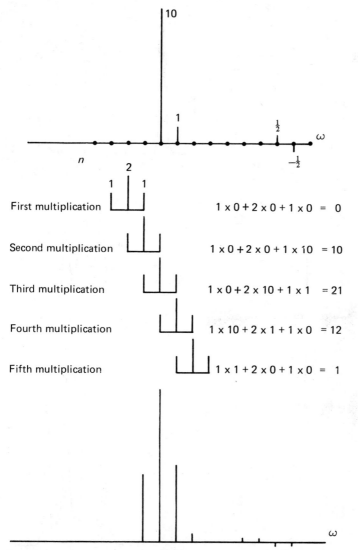

Figure 5.8   Demonstrating the convolution of a sharp spectral line consisting of two numbers, 10,1, by the function 1,2,1. This is strictly a triangular function but approximates a simple Lorenzian line. The function is moved through the data and at each position the numbers in the function are multiplied by the corresponding numbers in the data, summed and stored elsewhere to give a line which is a mixture of the two functions and is broadened. The way the function spreads out and attenuates the two noise spikes $\frac{1}{2}$, $-\frac{1}{2}$, is also shown.

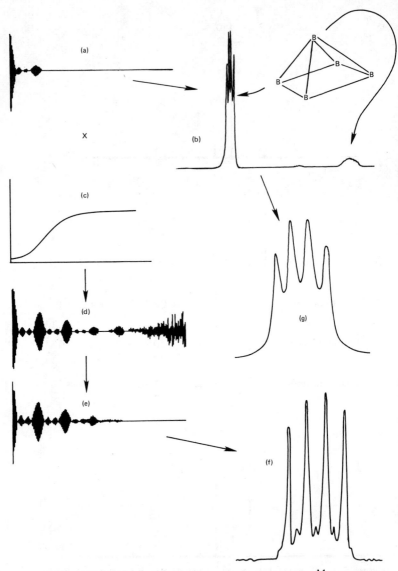

Figure 5.9   An example of resolution enhancement. The ^{11}B spectrum of the borane B_5H_9 is simplified if the protons are decoupled (see Chapter 7) and consists of a quartet due to the four basal boron atoms spin coupled to the apical boron. The apical boron gives a broad, unresolved resonance and we will not consider thus further. Some 18.8% of the apical boron atoms will be the isotope ^{10}B with $I = 3$ and so 18.8% of the basal resonance should be a septet. This is obscured by the more intense quartet due to those molecules with ^{11}B at the apex,

likely to be some break through of the pulse power into the data. In this case it may be helpful to attenuate decreasingly the first few points of data.

It is also possible to devise functions which have the opposite effect to that of exponential multiplication, namely to enhance the resolution, though they inevitably also degrade the signal to noise ratio. They are nevertheless being used more and more since they facilitate the interpretation of spectra and allow fine structure to be separated from overlying broad resonances or even show up features which normally are not observable. They aim ideally at producing a non-decaying FID and so start with a rising exponential of the same time constants as the decay of the FID. Unfortunately the noise present does not decay with time and so its intensity is much increased in the tail of the FID, hence the poor signal to noise ratio. Further, the noise can very quickly reach the value where it fills the memory words and the signal cannot then be registered and the transform becomes very distorted. Thus the function used has to rise only a limited amount and then stay constant or decrease again to minimize the noise. As a result, the FID decay is no longer exponential and the line-shape is no longer Lorenzian. It contains a Gaussian component, and indeed the process has been called a Lorenzian–Gaussian transformation. Unfortunately, Gaussian lines, while narrower at the base than Lorenzian ones, are thicker at the tip and so some of the benefit of the line narrowing processes is lost due to this transformation. In other words, the noise limits what we can achieve and it is essential to start with a low noise FID for useful improvement to be possible. An example of resolution enhancement is given in Fig. 5.9 and Fig. 5.10 compares the Lorenzian and Gaussian

---

whose lines overlap quite badly. The resolution needs to be improved if we are to observe the underlying septet. The FID collected from the sample is shown in (a) and the resulting spectrum in (b). A copy of the FID is multiplied, point by point, by the function (c) $1000/(999e^{-15n/4096} + 1)$, where n is the memory point within the 4K of memory used. This gives the FID (d) where the large increase in the noise will be observed. Only the first 2K is displayed in the figure and the second 2K is even more noisy. The noise is then reduced by a suitable function which leaves the signal part of the FID untouched − a Gaussian curve as in Fig. 5.10c for instance − to give a clean and much more slowly decaying FID (e). This transforms to give the spectrum (f) where three lines of the septet can now be observed, the other four being lost in the skirts of the two central lines of the quartet. The improvement in resolution can be seen by comparing (g), (an expanded plot of the quartet in (b)) and (f). (Reproduced with permission from Akitt (1978) *J. Mag. Res.*, **32**, 311.)

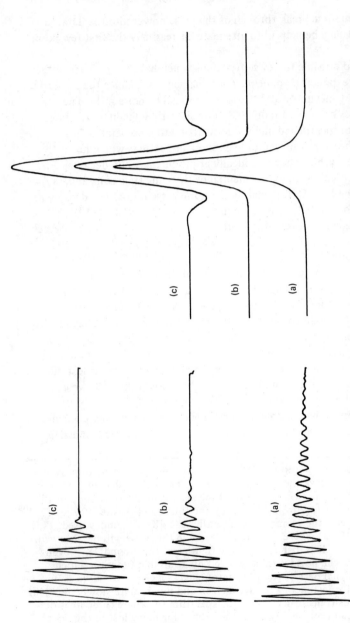

Figure 5.10 Three FIDs and their Fourier transforms. (a) An exponential decay gives a Lorenzian line with sharp top but broad skirts. (b) A Gaussian decay $I_n = I_0 e^{-(nT)^2}$ gives a Gaussian line with very narrow skirts but a thickened top. The rather more rapid decay which occurs early in the FID 'squares off' the base of the peak. (c) A super Gaussian decay $I_n = I_0 e^{-(nT)^4}$ introduces waves to each side of the peak and the top remains thick. Obviously, in the equation $I_0 = I_n e^{-(nT)^p}$, if p is very large we get a square wave decay and the transform is a sinc curve.

FIDs and their transforms. We should also note that the transform of the function shown in Fig. 5.9c is one positive point and a broad negative line underneath it. In other words we can think of this function as being the difference between a non-decaying FID (infinitely narrow line) and a rapidly decaying FID (broad negative line). Thus we see why it is also possible to carry out resolution enhancement by subjecting a copy of an FID to a substantial decaying exponential multiplication and then subtracting this from the original FID. Many procedures are now available for resolution enhancement though they have to be used with care since the final spectra are bound to contain both negative troughs and flanking wiggles to the peaks introduced by the functions used, and these can in extreme cases be mistaken for hidden peaks.

5.3   The Fourier transform

Equation 4.11 for the relationship between time and frequency domains is

$$F(\omega) = \int_{-\infty}^{\infty} f(t) \, (\cos \omega t - i \sin \omega t) \mathrm{d}t$$

It can be shown that it is valid to replace the continuous functions by discrete ones such as we collect in a computer, i.e. we can replace the integral symbols by summations, and can carry out a valid transform in a computer. The process of Fourier transformation can be thought of as carrying out a series of convolutions of the data by sine and cosine functions of all possible frequencies. If there is a frequency present equal to one of these then the convolution gives a value, and nothing in its absence. This would obviously be a very time consuming process and would require a vast amount of computer memory to store all the intermediate data needed. Fortunately, Cooley and Tukey have shown that provided all the data are contained in a memory with a number of locations equal to a power of 2 (1024, 2048, 4096, . . . etc. or in computer jargon, 1K, 2K, 4K, . . . etc. memory locations) then the process can be factorized in such a way as to remove many redundant multiplications and can be carried out in the data memory and using only a few extra locations to store numbers temporarily. The process is thus fast, times of only 5 to 20 s being required to transform an 8K block of data (8K = 8192). The existence of the Cooley–Tukey algorithm and of minicomputers were both necessary before FT NMR became a commercial possibility.

The sine and cosine convolutions produce, in effect, the two components of the nuclear magnetization in phase with and normal to B_1, and these are kept separate in the memory. The final result of the transform is thus two spectra which should in principle be the absorption and dispersion spectra. This assumes that the B_1 signal fed to the phase sensitive detector is exactly in Phase with B_1, a condition which it is very hard to realize in practice. Thus the two sets of spectra contain a mixture of dispersion and absorption. In addition we cannot be sure that we have started to collect data immediately after the B_1 pulse has ended; indeed, to avoid breakthrough we may have purposely delayed the collection of data, commonly by one dwell time. This means that the starting point for each frequency component differs since each type of nuclear magnet will have precessed by a different amount by the time data collection starts, their phases are different and the degree of admixture of the two spectra varies across the spectral width. The two components thus have to be separated, a procedure known as phase correction, which is an essential part of FT spectroscopy. The two halves of the sets of spectra are weighted and mixed according to the formulae below:

$$\text{new disp} = (\text{old disp})\cos \theta - (\text{old abs})\sin \theta$$
$$\text{new abs} = (\text{old abs})\cos \theta + (\text{old disp})\sin \theta$$

where abs means one half of the data and disp the other. The multiplication is carried out point by point through the data and θ is adjusted until one line is correctly phased, i.e. purely absorption in one half of memory and purely dispersion in the other half. This has to be done by trial and error monitoring the progress of the correction on the computer memory display screen. If not all the lines are then correctly phased, then it is necessary to repeat the correction but allow θ to vary linearly as a function of position in memory. It is best to arrange that $\theta = 0$ for the correctly phased line and allow it to vary to either side. This second process is then continued until all the lines are correctly phased. Attempts have been made to write automatic programs to carry out this rather tedious process but these have never been universally successful and the two stage process has always to be carried out by manual trial and error. The process is illustrated in Fig. 5.11.

Sometimes it happens that it is not possible to make a perfect phase correction. This may arise because the behaviour of the spin system is

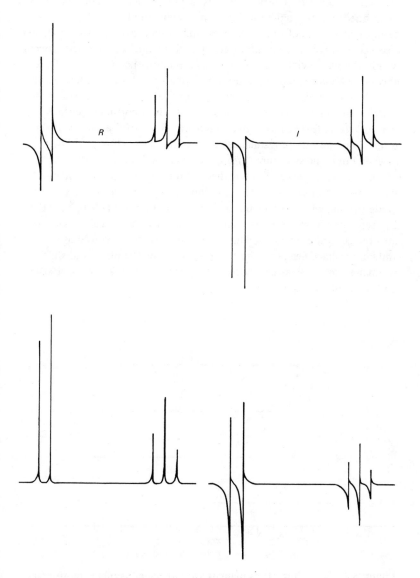

Figure 5.11   Phase correction. The upper pair of spectra are the two results of the transform operation, R and I, with scrambled phase of the lines of the AB_2 spectrum. A two parameter phase correction gives the purely absorption spectrum in one half and the purely dispersion form in the other.

affected by the way the spectrum has been obtained — we have already mentioned that too rapid pulsing if spin–spin coupling is present may result in distortion of line intensities, and in such a case phase anomalies also occur. If we have not arranged that all the nuclear resonances occur within the sweepwidth covered by the computer then those which are above the Nyquist frequency are out of phase with the rest. Similarly, resonances on either side of the B_1 carrier frequency will contribute to the FID though with different phase. It is thus important to ensure that all resonances occur on one side or the other of the carrier. If this is not done then those resonances outside the range chosen will be reflected into the spectrum through the 'mirrors' formed by the limits of the computer sweep. This is called folding or aliasing. The chemical shifts and phases will be wrong, and indeed the phase anomalies assist in identifying when a spectrum is folded. Provision is made to vary the B_1 frequency over a range so that it can be set to bring a given sample into the computer window. Thus we ensure that the two folding ambiguities have been avoided by observing how the phase and shift anomalies vary with sweepwidth and B_1 frequency. Spectra illustrating both sorts of folding are shown in Fig. 5.12.

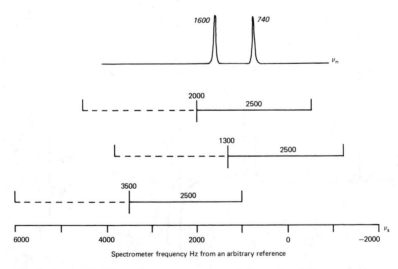

Figure 5.12   Folding of resonances around the ends of the computer memory 'window'. The spectrum consists of two resonances at 1600 and 740 Hz on an arbitrary scale related to the spectrometer frequency (13.8 MHz in this case for the ^{2}H nucleus). To set up correctly we place the spectrometer frequency to the high frequency side of both resonances, 2000 Hz in this case, and obtain an easily phase correctable

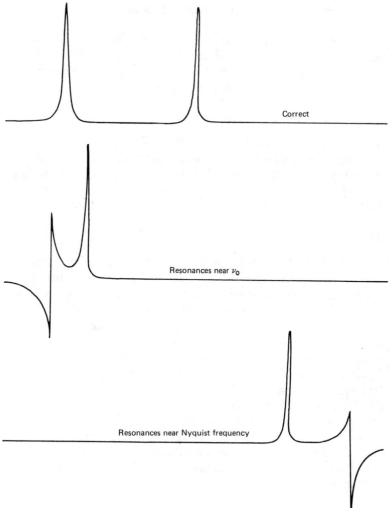

Correct

Resonances near ν_0

Resonances near Nyquist frequency

doublet, provided that the spectral width is large enough to accommodate the doublet; 2500 Hz being chosen in this case. If we reduce the spectrometer frequency to 1300 Hz, between the two lines, they appear at 300 and 440 Hz, close to the low frequency end of the scan, conventionally on the left. The phase of one line is now altered. We obtain the same effect if we alter the frequency so that the Nyquist frequency is between the lines. Here they appear at 600 and 260 Hz. The phase difference between the normal and folded lines depends upon the phase setting of the B_1 feed to the phase sensitive detector. A normal spectrum is obtained if ν_s is set to the low frequency side of the doublet but the lines are now reversed.

5.4   Manipulations in the frequency domain

Once we have the fully phase corrected spectrum in memory we now have to extract from it the information that we require. We will also need to make some sort of permanent record. Again, the computer allows us to carry out a variety of processes.

5.4.1   Data printout

This scans the spectrum to detect the lines, or at least those greater than the noise level by a certain amount, and then works out their frequency and chemical shift. The line due to a standard substance may be assigned a value zero so that the output then is a fully calibrated spectrum (Fig. 5.13). There many variations possible on this theme.

5.4.2   Integration

The initial intensity of an FID is proportional to the number of nuclei contributing to that signal and this transforms as the area of the Lorenzian absorption. An integral of the spectrum (we always of course refer to the absorption spectrum) then will tell us how many nuclei contribute to a given line and can give us invaluable quantitive data about a molecule — in the absence of relaxation effects discussed in Chapter 4. The integration is carried out simply by adding the numbers in successive memory locations. Where there is no resonance this sum will remain constant and will increase in the region of any resonance. The integral then forms a series of steps rising at each resonance (Fig. 5.14). This assumes of course that the base-line of the spectrum is at zero volts. In general this will not be true and means has to be provided to move the spectrum up or down in memory during integration. It is also possible to print out numerical integral figures though these may contain a base-line error.

5.4.3   Expansion

The typical oscilloscope screen is rather small to be able to observe much detail and it is often necessary to be able to expand part of the spectrum so as to see if there are, for instance, any small splittings.

5.4.4   Plotting data

This is achieved using an *XY* recorder driven by the computer. Digital to analogue converters read the numbers in memory to give a *Y*

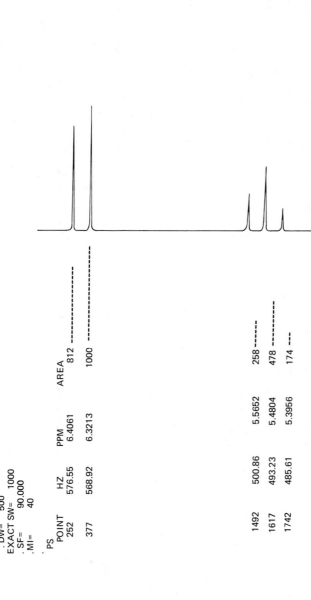

```
    . DW=    500
EXACT SW=   1000
  . SF=    90.000
  . MI=       40
  .
 PS
   POINT      HZ      PPM      AREA
    252     576.55   6.4061     812  -------------

    377     568.92   6.3213    1000  -------------




   1492     500.86   5.5652     258  -------
   1617     493.23   5.4804     478  -----------
   1742     485.61   5.3956     174  ----
```

Figure 5.13   An example of a computer printout placed beside the spectrum. The computer requires that an instruction be a two letter code. DW allows the dwell time to be inserted and the computer then calculates and prints the sweepwidth. SF allows the spectrometer frequency to be inserted and is used to calculate the chemical shift. MI is a minimum integral which causes the calculation to skip any small peaks of noise. PS causes the printout calculation to be carried out and list the memory address where the peak maximum is to be found, its frequency, its chemical shift, a number proportional to an integral and a dashed line proportional in height to the resonance. Each line is spaced out on approximately the same scale as the spectrum and this allows a comparison to be made easily between the printout and spectrum, which is invaluable if many lines are present. Note that the sum of areas is correct for an AB_2 spectrum.

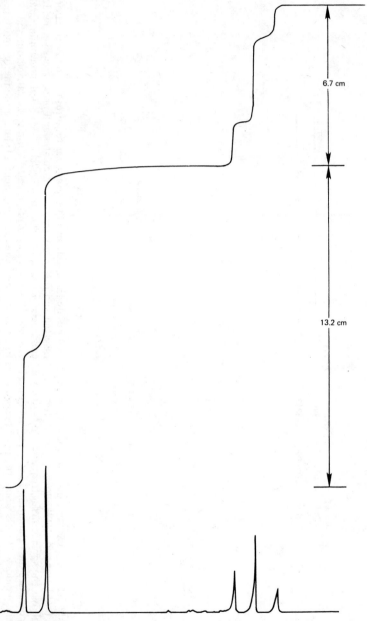

6.7 cm

13.2 cm

Figure 5.14   A spectrum and its integral. The heights of the two steps are closely in the ratio required for an AB_2 spectrum, 2:1.

deflection and a voltage relative to the memory location to give the X deflection. A sweep through the memory therefore allows the spectrum in memory to be drawn on paper. In addition the integral can be drawn, and the expanded sections, if necessary. Means are also provided to calibrate the paper. The spectrum (or, more likely, the FID) may also be stored in numerical form on disk or tape for future reference, though this is an expensive technique and can only be used to cover a limited period.

5.5   Continuous wave (CW) spectroscopy

Virtually all NMR spectrometers used for chemical work up to about 1970 were CW spectrometers and FT spectroscopy has developed since that time because of the pressing need to obtain ^{13}C spectra routinely at natural abundance and aided by the technical developments mentioned above. The technique in principle uses a weak, infinitely long, infinitely selective pulse — a continuous wave. This can only cause precession of the spin vectors at one point in the spectrum and so the B_1 frequency has to be swept slowly through the spectral width and the M_{xy} magnetization detected and recorded directly as the absorption mode spectrum on an XY recorder whose X axis is swept synchronously with the B_1 frequency. No computer is required so that the system is simpler and cheaper than an FT system though its sensitivity is much less, principally because so much of the sweep time is spent searching areas where there are no resonances.

The level of the B_1 field is set so as to avoid tipping the nuclear vectors too far and is determined by the relaxation time T_1, and the time taken to traverse the lines and hence the sweep rate. The method is applied today only to the most receptive nuclei (^1H, ^{19}F particularly). It has certain advantages over the FT method and only a small portion of the total spectrum need be examined so that dynamic range is much less of a problem. Neither is the resolution limited by the memory size of the computer. It has the disadvantage though that since the B_1 transmitter is on all the time this interferes with the nuclear signal and adds noise and base-line instability. These are minimized by modulating the magnetic field by passing an AC current through coils in the magnet gap around the sample. If we chose a frequency of 4000 Hz then the nuclear frequencies are modulated at this frequency and the signal can then be carried by the resulting side bands via a capacitor which blocks the low frequency variations causing instability. The sidebands each consist of a full spectrum and the modulation frequency has to be larger than the spectral width.

The frequency sweep has one consequence which is not observed in FT spectrometers. When $\mathbf{B}_1$ traverses a resonance, it creates magnetization M_{xy} precessing at the nuclear frequency which can only become of significant intensity at resonance, but which will retain significant intensity for a time of T_2^* afterwards. The $\mathbf{B}_1$ frequency changes continuously during this time and diverges from the nuclear frequency and so beats with it via the phase sensitive detector as the two go in and out of phase. The resonance is thus followed by a transient wiggle whose frequency of oscillation increases as the $\mathbf{B}_1$ and nuclear frequencies diverge. The decay constant of the wiggles is related to T_2^* though it is shorter than this because of the changing frequency and the effect of the RC filters present (Fig. 4.10). They are nevertheless a very useful phenomenon and are used universally to set up the homogeneity of the magnetic field by observing a sharp resonance and adjusting the shim currents until a smooth, prolonged exponential decay is obtained.

5.6   Time sharing spectrometers

These devices are in a way a compromise between FT and CW spectrometers. The transmitter output is in the form of weak, fairly long pulses at a repetition rate of say 4 kHz and the receiver is on only when the transmitter is off (Fig. 5.15). This gives, effectively, CW operation

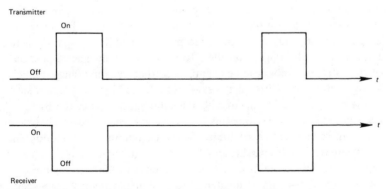

Figure 5.15   Receiver/transmitter time sharing. The receiver is switched off just before the transmitter is turned on, and remains off for a little while after the transmitter is turned off.

without the base-line instabilities. There is no need to modulate the magnetic field since the transmitter pulse modulation provides the sideband frequencies which can carry the signal. This means that the system is compatible with an FT device so that we can have two spectrometers associated with one magnet. Thus these devices, which are relatively simple, are used in conjunction with FT spectrometers to provide a final stage of stabilization using a nuclear resonance in the sample other than the one to be observed — often the deuterium in a deuterated solvent. The device is used in two ways. A small triangular repetitive sweep is applied temporarily to the magnetic field and the deuterium is observed in the absorption mode as its resonance is traversed repeatedly. We observe a signal followed by wiggles and can use this to set up the magnetic field homogeneity. We then switch off the field sweep and turn our attention to the dispersion signal produced by the solvent. This has the property that at resonance the output is zero, but if drift of field or frequency occurs, either a negative or positive output is obtained, the sign depending upon the direction of drift, and we can use this output to provide a correction voltage to alter the magnetic field until the output is again zero (Fig. 5.16). Thus the frequency and field are locked together indefinitely and we can in

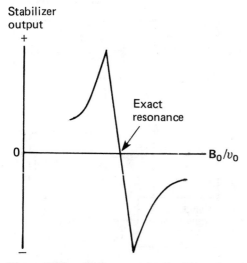

Figure 5.16   A resonance in the dispersion mode can be used to stabilize an NMR spectrometer. At exact resonance the output is zero but if drift occurs it becomes either positive or negative. The output can be used to provide a correction to the magnetic field which reverses the drift until the exact resonance position is regained.

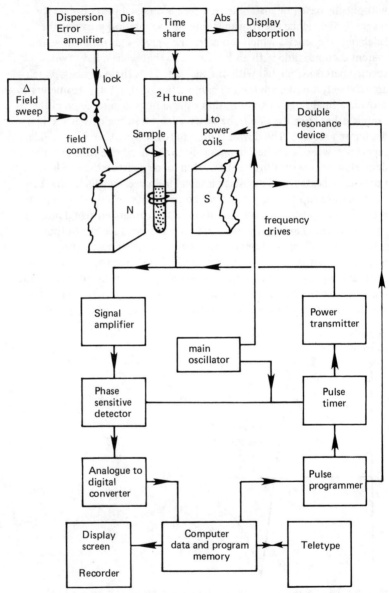

Figure 5.17   A full FT system.

principle accumulate as many FIDs in memory as we wish, 100 000 being quite feasible though the number is always kept as small as possible since there is very often a queue of people waiting to use any given spectrometer. It is of course necessary that the frequency of the lock device is derived from the FT drive frequency, otherwise they could vary independently. The lock then keeps the ratio B_0/ν_0 constant and is known as a field-frequency lock.

5.7   A modern system

The various parts of a complete FT spectrometer system are shown on the block diagram of Fig. 5.17. This summarizes much of what has been said in this chapter but also includes a double resonance device which we will need in Chapter 7. This is a third transmitter which can provide power at the frequency of other nuclear isotopes in the sample, pulsed or continuous, and so affect their behaviour and modify the response of the nuclei observed.

6
The Sample

An NMR experiment involves a highly sophisticated instrument capable of resolving resonances and making measurements to a few parts in 10^9. (This is equivalent to comparing the lengths of two steel rods each 1 km long to within one thousandth part of 1 mm.) One must, therefore, accept the responsibility of preparing a sample which will not degrade the spectrometer performance. However any sample placed in the magnet gap will distort the magnetic field. Fortunately, the distortion occurs externally to a cylindrical sample and the field remains homogeneous within it except at the ends, though its magnitude is changed by an amount which depends both on the shape of the sample and upon the bulk magnetic susceptibility of the tube glass and of the sample itself. Imperfections in the glass, variations in wall thickness, variations in diameter, or curvature of the cylinder along its length all lead to degredation of the field homogeneity within the sample with consequent line broadening. For this reason high precision bore sample tubes are always used for NMR. Since solid particles distort the field around them, suspended solids must also be filtered from the liquid sample prior to measurement.

6.1   Standardization

We have shown that chemical shifts are invariably measured relative to a standard of some sort. There are three ways of standardizing a resonance, namely:

6.1.1   Internal standardization

The standard substance is dissolved in the sample solution and its resonance appears in the spectrum. This method has the advantage that the magnetic field is exactly the same at sample and standard molecules. The standard must be chosen so as not to obscure sample resonances and also must be inert to the sample. Internal standardization is the method normally used and the two techniques below are used only in special cases.

The main disadvantage of the method is that weak interactions with the solvent produce small chemical shifts which are difficult to predict and which reduce the accuracy of the measurements by an unknown amount. These shifts are said to arise from solvent effects.

6.1.2   External standardization

The standard is sealed into a capilliary tube which is placed coaxially within the sample tube. The main disadvantages of the method is that since the volume magnetic susceptibilities of the sample and standard will differ by several tenths of a ppm, the magnetic fields in each will be different and a correction will have to be made for this. Since the volume susceptibilities of solutions are often not known these must be measured, so that a single shift determination becomes quite difficult if accurate work is required. The magnitude of the correction depends upon the sample shape and is zero for spherical samples so that this disadvantage can be minimized by constructing special concentric spherical sample holders. The method is used with very reactive samples or with samples where lack of contamination is important.

Because the capilliary holding the standard distorts the magnetic field around it, the field homogeneity in the annular outer part of the sample is destroyed. This can be restored by spinning, which is essential with this type of standardization. Distorted capilliaries can even then degrade the resolution and if there is any asymmetry in the annular region this will be averaged by spinning to give a field different in value from the true average, i.e. a small shift error will result. The method is nevertheless the only one suitable for measuring solvent shifts. Fig. 6.1 shows spectra obtained from coaxial sample tubes.

6.1.3   Substitution

In this case the sample and standard are placed in separate tubes of the same size and are recorded separately in the order standard, sample, standard so that if there is no lock available any field drift that occurs during the measurements can be allowed for. If the samples both contain a compound which can provide a lock then their frequencies

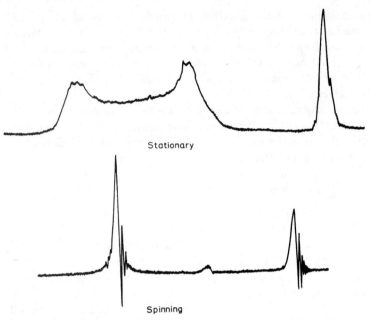

Stationary

Spinning

Figure 6.1   The field in the annular portion of a coaxial sample tube is distorted and in a stationary tube gives a broad twin-horned resonance. The capilliary resonance is the sharp one to high field of the annular signal. The distance between the horns is a measure of the volume magnetic susceptibility of the fluid in the annulus. If the tube is spun the molecules in the annulus experience an average field and a sharp singlet results. (^{1}H spectra of aqueous solutions.)

can be compared directly in two measurements though with the same reservations as for the previous technique above. The locking system does of course allow standardization of a spectrum of one isotope species using another, either that of the lock, or of a third via the lock substance. In fact today many spectra are recorded for relatively dilute samples in deuterated lock solvents so that all are in effect referred to the same internal secondary standards. In the majority of cases therefore, solvent effects and susceptibility changes are ignored unless particularly accurate comparitive work is required. Indeed, this is the method commonly used for referring all but proton and carbon spectra, where TMS is usually added to the sample.

Spinning side bands are often seen in spectra flanking the more intense lines and spaced equally to either side of them. They are only seen when the sample is spinning and their spacing from the central line depends on the speed of spinning. They arise because the magnetic field homogeneity is not perfect so that an individual nucleus, as it moves in the circular path impressed by the spinning, experiences a regularly fluctuating field. Their resonance width is reduced but their frequency is modulated and a series of sidebands are produced separated by the spinning frequency. These become weaker if the spinning speed is increased though the speed is limited by the tendency for the sample to be thrown up the wall of the tube and spoil the homogeneity, unless a plug is pushed down the tube to confine the sample.

6.2   Solvent effects

The solvent shift effects mentioned under internal standardization, while a nuisance to those interested simply in structure determination, are of interest in their own right, since they tell us something about the weak interactions which occur between solvent and solutes. The effect is particularly large for aromatic solvents or where specific interactions occur. The chemical shifts of a number of substances relative to TMS in a series of solvents are given in Table 6.1

Table 6.1   Internal chemical shifts δ of solutes in different solvents.

Solvent	Solvent				
	$CDCl_3$	$(CD_3)_2SO$	Pyridine	Benzene	CF_3COOH
Acetone $(CH_3)_2CO$	2.17	2.12	2.00	1.62	2.41
Chloroform $CHCl_3$	7.27	8.35	8.41	6.41	7.25
Dimethyl sulphoxide $(CH_3)_2SO$	2.62	2.52	2.49	1.91	2.98
Cyclohexane C_6H_{12}	1.43	1.42	1.38	1.40	1.47

The variation in δ between solvents of course contains contributions from the solvent effect on both solute and standard. The table nevertheless is useful in indicating the existence of certain interactions involving the solutes. Thus the high field shifts obtained in the aromatic solvent benzene and for all solutes but chloroform in the aromatic solvent pyridine are obvious. Even the relatively inert cyclohexane is shifted upfield by 0.05 ppm. This arises because solutes tend to spend a larger amount of time face on to the disc shaped aromatic molecules and so on average are shifted high field by the ring current anisotropy. The magnitude of the effect depends upon molecular shape and is also increased if there is any tendency for polar groups in the molecule to interact with the aromatic π-electrons. Fig. 6.2 shows that the larger proportion of the space around a benzene molecule suffers ring current screening.

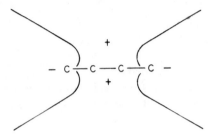

Figure 6.2   Volumes of space around a benzene ring where a proton may be screened (+) or descreened (−). There is a greater likelihood on average that the benzene will approach a solute molecule face on and therefore screen its protons. (After Johnson and Bovey (1958) *J. Chem. Phys.*, **29**, 1012.) The ring is shown edge-on.

In the case of complex solutes each type of proton in the molecule suffers a solvent shift but because the proximity of each to solvent depends upon the shape of the molecule, each suffers a different solvent shift. For this reason a complex solute may have quite different spectra in chloroform and benzene and this fact is used to help simplify and interpret complex spectra. Fig. 6.3 gives an example.

Figure 6.3   Part of the 90 MHz proton spectrum of a dithioglycoside dissolved in carbon tetrachloride or in benzene. The protons directly bonded to the $C_5 S$ ring are depicted by their serial number only on the inset formula. In carbon tetrachloride the 2- and 4-proton resonances overlap but become well separated in benzene solution.

The dependence of the vicinal coupling constant upon the dihedral angle between protons is also well illustrated in this spectrum. H_2 is coupled to two protons giving a doublet of doublets. It is coupled to H_1 by 10.6 Hz. Both protons are axial, the dihedral angle is about 170° and the coupling is near the maximum (see Fig. 3.7). H_2 is also coupled to H_3 by 2.6 Hz. The coupling is much smaller since one proton is axial and the other equational to give a dihedral angle near 60°.

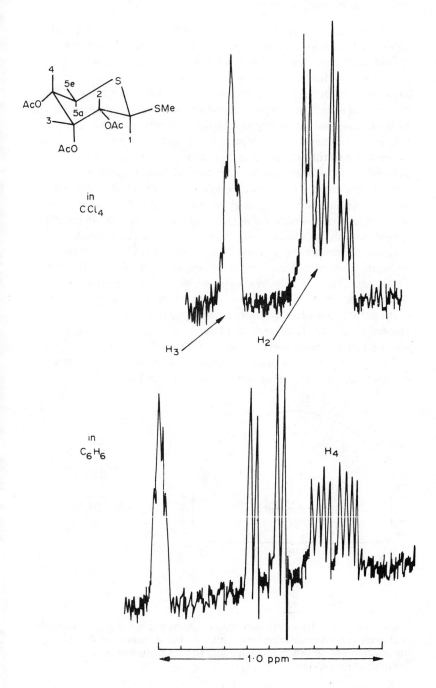

in
CCl₄

H₃   H₂

in
C₆H₆

H₄

|← 1·0 ppm →|

Chloroform as a solute suffers considerable solvent shifts. The pure liquid is self-associated by hydrogen bonding but upon progressive dilution in an inert solvent the proportion of hydrogen-bonded molecules is reduced and its resonance is shifted 0.29 ppm upfield. The shifts noted in the table are in excess of this and we must consider the existence of several other types of interaction. Thus specific interactions with the Lewis bases dimethyl-sulphoxide and pyridine result in low field shifts. In the case of pyridine this implies a preference for an edge on approach to the aromatic ring and therefore some ring current deshielding. In benzene, on the other hand, hydrogen bonding is reduced, and there is probably face-wise interaction of the chloroform with the benzene π-electrons. Both processes tend to increase the screening so that the chloroform is shifted strongly upfield. In addition, the chloroform molecule is polar and its dipole electric field will polarize the surrounding solvent by an amount related to the solvent dielectric constant ϵ. The molecule, shown as the dipole M in Fig. 6.4, can be regarded as residing in a cavity whose walls become charged. This induced charge gives rise to an electric field, R, which is called the reaction field and which will also produce chemical shifts of the chloroform solute. Thus some of the variation observed in Table 6.1 will originate from differences in solvent dielectric constant.

The effect of changes in solvent dielectric constant can be clearly demonstrated by the relative solvent shifts obtained for the 4- and

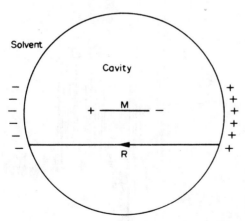

Figure 6.4   A polar solute molecule polarizes the surrounding solvent and generates an electric reaction field, R. The direction of R follows the motion of the solute molecule and thus can cause electric field induced chemical shifts.

2-protons of 3, 5-dimethylpyridine (3, 5-lutidine). This molecule produces an electric field as shown in Fig. 6.5. The field R has different components along the carbon—hydrogen bonds at the 2 and 4 positions, having its full value along the bond to the 4-hydrogen while it is nearly zero along that to the 2-hydrogen. One would therefore expect that the 4-hydrogen would move low field as the solvent dielectric constant was increased since its electrons can be pulled along the bond away from the hydrogen, whereas the 2-hydrogen should be much less affected. Since the two atoms reside in the same fairly simple molecule one can have some confidence that specific effects and anisotropy shifts will be similar for both protons and that the observed solvent shifts between them arise primarily from the electric reaction field. The 2- (and 6-) protons resonate low field of the 4-proton. As solvents of higher dielectric constant are employed the 4-proton resonance is observed to approach that of the 2- and 6-protons so moving low field as predicted (Table 6.2).

Two further contributions to solvent shifts are also usually considered. One arises from the van der Waals interactions and is

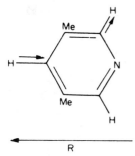

Figure 6.5   The reaction field of 3, 5-dimethyl pyridine has maximum effect along the bond to the 4-hydrogen and a small and opposite effect along the bonds to the 2- and 6-hydrogens. The chemical shift between the 4- and 2- (or 6-) hydrogens therefore depends upon solvent polariz-ability. The small arrows near the bonds indicate the direction of electron drift.

Table 6.2   The effect of solvent dielectric constant upon the 2, 4 shift

Solvent	C_6H_{12}	CCl_4	$CDCl_3$	Me_2CO	MeOH
ϵ	2.02	2.24	4.81	21.3	33.62
2, 4 shift ppm	1.04	0.97	0.95	0.84	0.70

responsible for vapour–liquid shifts of 0.1 to 0.5 ppm. The other arises in the case of external standardization and is due to bulk diamagnetic susceptibility differences between solvents. These susceptibility shifts can be comparable in magnitude with those due to the other effects and so must be considered in any interpretation of solvent shifts, but they do not of course arise from any chemical interaction.

The various contributions to the solvent shift δ_S can be summarized by a five-term equation:

$$\delta_S = \delta_B + \delta_A + \delta_E + \delta_H + \delta_W \tag{6.1}$$

where δ_B is the bulk susceptibility contribution, δ_A is the anisotropy contribution, δ_E is the reaction field contribution, δ_H is the contribution of hydrogen bonding and specific interactions, and δ_W is the van der Waals contribution.

7
Multiple Resonance Experiments

We have already seen that it is possible to subject a sample to more than one radio frequency field and obtain both a lock signal and a diagnostic signal, usually from nuclei situated in different molecules in the sample. In Fig. 5.17 we indicated that it is possible to subject a sample to further irradiation and we shall now discuss the effect of this, concentrating upon what happens when one type of nucleus in a molecule is irradiated at its resonant frequency while another is being observed, in the same molecule. We find that certain of the observed signals are perturbed by this procedure and that the nuclei affected are coupled in some way to the irradiated nuclei. This procedure is known as a double resonance experiment and has allowed the performance of some most elegant NMR investigations of chemical systems. The number of different nuclei irradiated is not limited theoretically and so triple, quadruple, . . . resonance experiments are also carried out though they become increasingly complex both in terms of interpretation and instrumentation. The double resonance experiment can be homonuclear, i.e. among like nuclei which are chemically shifted, or heteronuclear, i.e. one species is observed while another is irradiated. These two cases are differentiated by writing, e.g. $^{19}F\{^{19}F\}$ or $^{13}C\{^{1}H\}$ respectively, where the irradiation is applied to the nucleus in the brackets and the other is observed. This irradiation, which we shall call B_2, may be a weak, with a monochromatic frequency, or strong and monochromatic (which nevertheless had bandwidth because of the Lorenzian shape of NMR resonances), or it may be given a large bandwidth by some form of pseudo random or noise modulation which produces an even spread of sidebands over several thousand Hz. B_2 can also be applied continuously or in the form of pulses at different times during the experiment which allows the study of different facets of a system. Multiple irradiation can also be associated with FT or CW spectrometers and the techniques used are then different as indeed is the range of experiments which may be carried out. Nuclei can be coupled in several ways: via the bonds, i.e. spin—spin coupling; via chemical exchange; or via the through-space relaxation field. Each coupling path leads to different double resonance effects and we shall discuss them separately.

7.1   Double resonance and spin—spin coupling

The double irradiating field is applied in the same way as the B_1 field, i.e. in coils which give a rotating magnetic vector. If B_2 is the magnitude of the irradiating field and γ is the magnetogyric ratio of the nucleus irradiated, then we can define a frequency ν_2 such that $\nu_2 = \gamma B_2/2\pi$.

Irradiating field strength is usually expressed in terms of ν_2, and may be of the order of one or less Hz, when single lines in spin multiplets may be selectively irradiated without affecting other lines (low power or tickling irradiation), or may be several Hz when all the lines in a multiplet may be affected simultaneously (high power irradiation). In this case $\nu_2 \approx J$.

If we use low power double irradiation then we find that in order to observe any effect we have to tune our B_2 transmitter close to the frequency of an individual line, the lower the power the more exact must be the tuning. The rotating component of B_2 is then stationary relative to the irradiated nuclei. We can think of it as causing a precession of the irradiated nuclei at frequency ν_2. If ν_2 is very low ($\nu_2 \approx 1/T_1$) then any precession is opposed by relaxation effects and all that occurs in effect is a steady flow of quantal spin transitions to the higher energy states. This means that the populations of the spin states associated with the transition irradiated are perturbed. What happens is depicted in Fig. 7.1, which shows a fragment of the cube diagram used to discuss the three spin system in Chapter 3, Fig. 3.15. Thus, if the transition A_2 is irradiated, the spin population of the upper energy state $--+$ will be increased and that of the lower energy state $+-+$ will be depleted. Since the population of the highest energy state $---$ is even smaller than that of $--+$ then the population difference involved in the C_4 transition is increased and its intensity increases. On the other hand, the population of $-++$ is greater than $--+$ and the intensity of B_2 decreases. The transitions associated with the lower

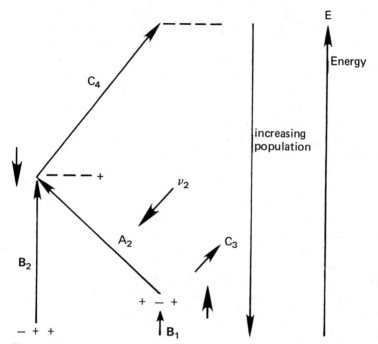

Figure 7.1   A fragment of the energy level diagram of Fig. 3.15 for
the three spin system illustrating the effect of weak irradiation of one
of the transitions A_2. This causes population changes in the two energy
levels involved due to absorption of energy, the short, triangular arrows
indicating the way the populations change. The result is to increase the
intensity of transitions C_4 and B_1 and to decrease that of transitions
B_2 and C_3.

energy level of A_2 also suffer change and C_3 decreases and B_1 increases.
The effect is often described as a generalized Overhauser effect. The
pairs of transitions are classified into progressive or regressive pairs.
The term progressive is used if there is a progressive increase in energy
from the lower end of one transition to the far end of the connected
one ($A_2 C_4$ in this case) and regressive if the two levels have the same
common highest or lowest energy level ($A_2 B_2$). Then we can say that
the intensity of the progressive transitions is increased by irradiation
and that of regressive transitions decreased.

This experiment can be carried out in either the CW or FT mode
and is called an INDOR (InterNuclear DOuble Resonance) or PSEUDO
INDOR experiment, respectively. In the CW mode, $\mathbf{B_2}$ is arranged to

be swept steadily through the spectral region while a single transition is monitored, i.e. B_1 is set at the tip of a resonance so that there is a continual output from the nuclei concerned. This is commonly registered on a recorder whose X axis is swept synchronously with the B_2 frequency. Every time B_2 attains the frequency of a connected transition, there is an intensity change which indicates whether it is a progressive or regressive transition. Four such transitions are observed for the three spin system and can be observed without interference from overlying resonances, it being sufficient to be able to resolve only the line monitored. The changes are quite small and the resulting spectra tend to be rather noisy. By using the FT mode, a better noise level can be obtained though the technique is different. A normal spectrum is obtained, without irradiation, and stored in part of data memory. A second spectrum is then run while one resonance is subjected to weak B_2 irradiation and collected in a second part of memory. Finally, the two spectra are subtracted in memory to leave only the parts of the spectrum which were affected by the irradiation. The two techniques are illustrated in Fig. 7.2. This technique of *difference spectroscopy* is much used in FT NMR though there is always the problem that the B_2 field may perturb the spectrum instrumentally. For this reason the normal spectrum is run with B_2 on, but tuned outside the spectral range.

The power of irradiation described above was of the order of a resonance line-width. If ν_2 is increased to a few line-widths, the Overhauser population changes still occur but are obscured by a new effect. The precession around ν_2 now appears to modulate the coupling to the other nuclei in the molecule and so splits a proportion of the lines into doublets of spacing ν_2. The lines affected are the same as in the previous case. Progressive and regressive transitions can be differentiated since the former are better resolved and can indeed have lines narrower than the magnetic field inhomogeneity. The technique is essentially a CW one and is known to the trade as a *tickling* experiment. It allows energy level diagrams to be set up for a system and gives rapidly information on the relative signs of coupling constants. Thus if a low field line of a multiplet is tickled and this leads to splitting in the high field part of one associated multiplet and the low field part of another, then the two coupling constants are of opposite sign.

A second and spectacular use of the low power technique is to obtain the spectra of nuclei which might not be observable with a given spectrometer. For instance, most spectrometers will be able to produce a proton spectrum of the ammonium ion NH_4^+, which is a 1:1:1 triplet,

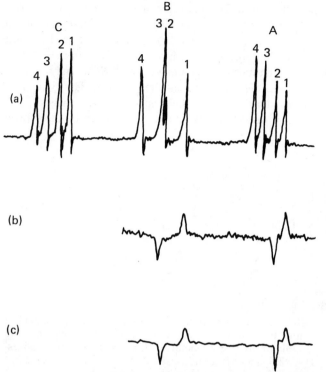

Figure 7.2   (a) The ^{1}H CW spectrum of 1,2-dibromopropionic acid at 100 MHz in deuteriobenzene. (b) The INDOR CW spectrum of 1,2-dibromopropionic acid at 100 MHz *monitoring* line C4. (c) The pseudo INDOR FT spectrum of 1,2-dibromopropionic acid at 100 MHz *irradiating* line C4. (Reproduced with permission from Feeney and Partington (1973) *J. Chem. Soc. Chem. Commun.*, 611).

but very few can produce the ^{14}N spectrum, which is a quintet. The proton spectrometer can be used to produce the ^{14}N quintet with the addition only of an auxiliary transmitter operating at the ^{14}N frequency. No ^{14}N receiver or sample coil replacement is required.

The experiment is carried out by adjusting the spectrometer so that it is continually tuned to one of the proton resonances. We obtain a constant spectrometer output from the protons. We then apply weak irradiation near the ^{14}N frequency using the auxiliary transmitter and sweep its frequency. Every time the frequency corresponds to one of the ^{14}N quintet lines, part of the proton line is split into a doublet and the intensity of the central line is reduced. Thus if we sweep the ^{14}N frequency and the recorder simultaneously we will observe a change in the spectrometer output every time a ^{14}N line is traversed and a quintet will be drawn out. The proportion split out depends upon the proportion of ^{1}H spin states contributing to the ^{14}N line and so the quintet is drawn with the correct intensities (Fig. 7.3). This type of experiment is also known as an INDOR experiment. It is a CW technique though it can be modified to be used with an FT instrument.

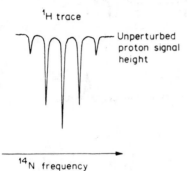

Figure 7.3   INDOR spectrum of the ^{14}N resonance of NH_4^+ in acidic solution obtained by observing one line of the proton resonance while sweeping a double irradiation transmitter through the ^{14}N resonances. $^1J(^{14}N-^1H) = 52.6$ Hz. (After Gillies and Randall (1971) *Progress in NMR Spectroscopy*, Vol. 6, p. 131, with permission.)

The two low power techniques have in common the fact that B_2 must be tuned accurately to a resonance for an effect to be observed. If v_2 is increased then its effective width becomes comparable with the whole spread of a multiplet. High power double irradiation thus need only be applied near the centre of a multiplet whether there is a line there or not and its effect is to split all the lines arising from a coupled nucleus. The splitting is asymmetric and the lines nearest the centre of the multiplet are most intense. As v_2 and the line splitting are increased the lines moving nearer to the centre of the multiplet crowd together while those moving away from the centre lose intensity. When v_2 is large enough all the intensity is at the centre of the multiplet and a singlet is observed. The irradiated nucleus is said to have been decoupled. The condition for this is that $v_2 \gg J$. The technique is used for the simplification of spectra and is most easily applied to the heteronuclear case where the nuclear frequencies are well separated, so that the powerful double resonance transmitter cannot interfere with the spectrometer receiver system. Like nuclei can be decoupled if their resonances are separated by a frequency very much larger than the coupling constant between them. In this case however, if an FT spectrometer is used, the B_2 signal would interfere with the nuclear response and swamp the receiver so that a time shared method is used in which the receiver and B_2 are never on simultaneously. Some experiments are outlined in Figs. 7.4, 7.5 and 7.6 and the homonuclear time shared experiment is described in Fig. 7.7.

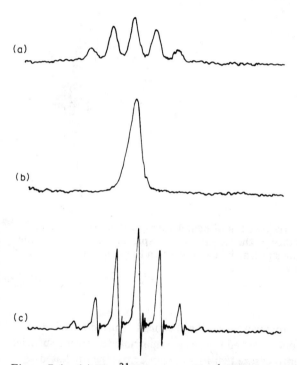

Figure 7.4   (a) The ^{31}P spectrum ($I = \frac{1}{2}$) of triethylphosphite $(CH_3CH_2O)_3P$. Both the methyl and the methylene protons are coupled to the phosphorus, the six methylene protons producing a septet and the methyls a decet. The P-to-methyl proton coupling is small and leads to unresolved broadening of the septet lines. The outer lines are lost in noise. (b) This is confirmed by irradiating the CH_2 methylene protons when only an unresolved decet remains due to the CH_3C-P interaction. (c) If instead the methyl resonance is irradiated, the septet due to coupling to the methylene protons becomes well resolved since the methyl protons responsible for the broadening are decoupled.

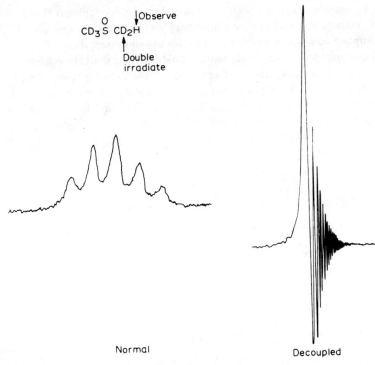

Figure 7.5   The ^{1}H spectrum of pentadeutero dimethyl sulphoxide. The proton resonance of the CD_2H group is split into a quintet by the two deuterons. The splitting is removed when the deuterium resonance is strongly irradiated.

If it is required to decouple all the chemically shifted nuclei of one species from the one observed it is often impossible to provide sufficient transmitter power to ensure that $\nu_2 \gg J$ right across the irradiated spectrum. In this case it is necessary to spread out the $\mathbf{B}_2$ frequency using noise modulation so that it has components at all frequencies in the spectral range. Such irradiation removes all spin–spin coupling and, for instance, in a $^{31}P\{^1H\}$ experiment, such as in Fig. 7.4, the ^{31}P spectrum then becomes a singlet, which obviously results in a very large improvement in signal to noise ratio. This feature is particularly useful for the less receptive nuclei and was used originally in $^{13}C\{^1H\}$ spectroscopy to ensure that each type of carbon gave an intense singlet resonance (Fig. 7.8).

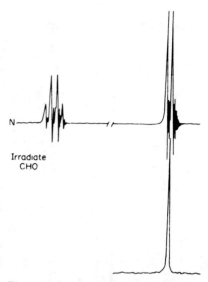

Irradiate
CHO

Figure 7.6   An example of high power homonuclear double irradiation. N shows the normal spectrum of acetaldehyde CH_3CHO and below it the spectrum of the methyl group run while the formyl proton was double irradiated. (Reproduced with permission from Bovey (1965) *Chem. and Eng. News*, 30 Aug, 118.)

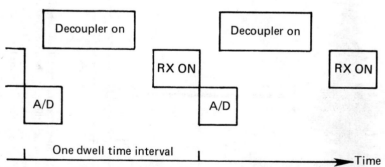

Figure 7.7   Time shared homonuclear FT decoupling. Three parts of the spectrometer have to be switched on and off independently though in a particular order. The receiver alone is switched on for sufficient time to establish an output (RX ON). This output is fed to the analogue to digital converter which starts to convert the voltage into a number at a precise time, set by the dwell time in use, and takes a finite time to make the conversion, 5 to 20 μs (A/D). The decoupler is switched on during the A/D conversion process and remains on until a little while before the receiver is switched on again. The effect of the decoupler may be modified by reducing the length of each pulse as required.

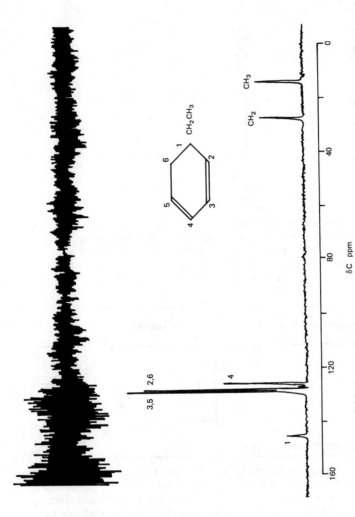

Figure 7.8   A carbon-13 spectrum in the FT mode of a solution of ethyl benzene in deuterio chloroform, $CDCl_3$, which is used also as deuterium lock. The ethyl benzene protons have been decoupled from the ^{13}C by broad band proton irradiation at 90 mHz and the spectrum represents the transform of 3000 accumulated transients at a spectrometer frequency of 22.62 mHz. No $^{13}C-^{13}C$ coupling is observed because most molecules will contain only one ^{13}C atom. The data were collected in 8K of memory at a rate of 88 transients per minute using a 40° pulse. The first 1K of the FID is

If the broad band modulation is not used then all the multiplets are affected differently. Any near the B_2 frequency will be decoupled but those further away still show coupling patterns, though the splitting observed is reduced. It is possible to tell in this case how many protons are coupled to a given carbon atom whereas with no decoupling the lines overlap too much to allow easy assignment. This information of course helps in the assignment of particular resonances to particular carbon atoms in the molecule. The frequency of irradiation which allows a certain multiplet to be decoupled tells us the frequency, and chemical shift, of the protons attached to that carbon. By carrying out several such experiments at different B_2 frequencies (known usually as offset frequencies) the way the apparent J varies for each type of carbon can be plotted and this allows a full connection to be made between the proton and carbon resonances (Fig. 7.9). This is known as an off resonance decoupling experiment.

It is in fact possible to control the value of apparent coupling observed quite precisely, and while this is not much used, the technique is illustrative in the present context. Broad band irradiation is applied in the form of pairs of pulses occurring during each dwell time period. Thus B_2 is switched on for a time t and causes all the protons to precess around B_2 is a certain direction. At the end of time t, the phase of the B_2 signal is changed by $180°$. This reverses the direction of the B_2 component around which the spins are precessing and so they now precess in the opposite direction. After a further time t they have returned to their original position and B_2 is switched off. This is repeated between each point in time where the signal is sampled, and in effect gives the protons an orientation which is an average of those taken during the pulses. The component of magnetization seen by the carbon nuclei is then less than its normal value so that J_r is less than the true J and is controlled by the proportion of time taken by the pulses (Fig. 7.10).

7.2   Through-space coupling via the relaxation field

The T_1 relaxation mechanism involves an exchange of energy between a nuclear system and the degrees of freedom of motion of the whole system which gives rise to the relaxation field. Energy transfer is slow and the relaxation times of spin $\frac{1}{2}$ nuclei are long. If, however, we strongly irradiate one group of nuclei using a double irradiation trans-mitter we grossly perturb the nuclear populations. The relaxation field

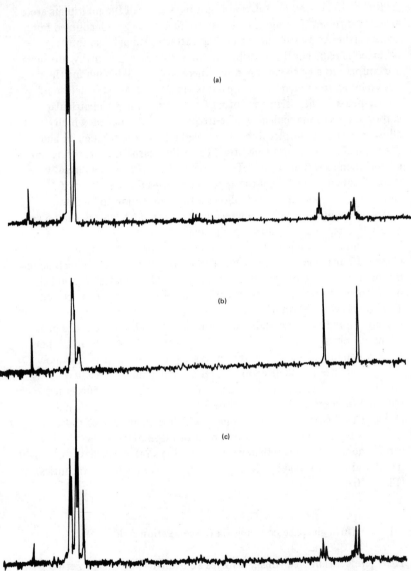

Figure 7.9   Off resonance proton decoupled carbon-13 FT spectra. The
spectra have been obtained in each case with strong irradiation in the
proton region with a continuous, unmodulated B_2 placed at different
points in the proton region. In (a) this was close to the phenyl protons
whose bonded carbons all give singlets as in Fig. 7.8, whereas the
ethyl group resonances show as a triplet and quartet of reduced

attempts to return the population to equilibrium and in so doing adsorbs much more energy than is normal from the irradiated nuclei. If other nuclei lie close in space to the irradiated nuclei then there is a chance that they will individually provide some of this energy and undergo nuclear transitions which will alter the populations of their spin states also. A change in their resonance intensity is observed and this feature can be used to determine conformations of organic molecules. The phenomenon is known as the Overhauser effect. It occurs in all double resonance experiments and small intensity changes are often observed in the various types of experiment described previously. An example of the use of the method to determine the conformation of a compound is given later.

The maximum value that the Overhauser effect can have is determined by the nature of the nuclear species involved. Since the phenomenon is controlled by relaxation processes, it falls off as r^{-6}, where r is the distance between the nuclei concerned, and so is important only if the nuclei are in close proximity. Provided the extreme narrowing condition is met, it does not depend upon operating frequency and is given by

$$(\eta_I^S)_{max} = \frac{\gamma_S}{2\gamma_I}$$

where I is the spin observed and S is that irradiated, and the γs are their magnetogyric ratios. In the homonuclear case η_{max} is just $\frac{1}{2}$, the maximum intensity observable is $1 + \frac{1}{2}$ of normal, and the effect is quite small. If the γ_s are very different, as will be the case if ^1H is irradiated and another nucleus observed, then the effect can be substantial since the perturbation of a large magnetic moment needs to strongly involve a smaller moment. Since γ can be negative (e.g. ^{15}N or

---

splitting. In (b) the proton frequency was moved into the alkyl region and the ethyl group now gives two singlets while the phenyl carbons appear as doublets of reduced splitting. In (c) the irradiation was moved outside the proton spectrum, past the alkyl region, and all the carbons show coupling to hydrogen (except, of course, the 4-carbon). The phenyl protons are furthest away from the B_2 frequency and so show the largest carbon–hydrogen splitting. The value of this residual splitting, J_r, is predictable and can be calculated from the formula:

$$\nu_{B_2} - \nu_H = J_r \gamma_{B_2} / 2\pi J$$

where J is the true C–H coupling constant, ν_{B_2} is the frequency of irradiation and ν_H is the corresponding proton frequency.

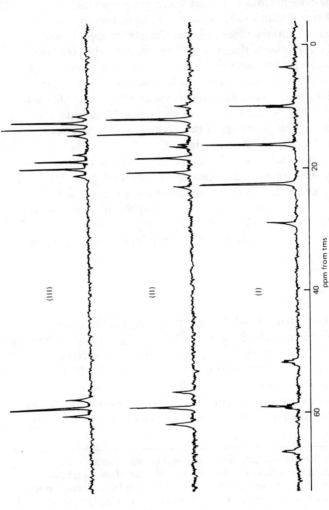

Figure 7.10   Scaling the ^{1}H—^{13}C coupling constants observed in the ^{13}C spectrum of ethyl acetate. (1) shows the spectrum without decoupling. The two CH$_3$ quartets overlap badly. Note also the small two bond J(C—H) in the ethyl group. (2) ^1J is reduced to 35.6% of its true value by irradiating the protons for 80 μs then changing the phase for a further 80 μs and then waiting 118 μs. The total time of the sequence is 278 μs, or one dwell time. The pulse is situated in the interval between taking samples of the signal. (3) ^1J reduced to 17.8% of its value by longer pulses of 100 μs and 78 μs waiting time. Note that the small two bond coupling is not now resolvable. (Reproduced with permission from Aue and Ernst (1978) *J. Mag. Res*, **31**, 533.)

^{29}Si), η_{max} can be negative also, leading to negative going signals if $\eta > 1$. A number of interfering factors ensure that the effect actually observed, η_{obs}, is often less than the theoretical. There can be two

Table 7.1   *Maximum nuclear Overhauser effects for several pairs of*
nuclei. (From Martin, Delpuech and Martin, *Practical NMR*
Spectroscopy, John Wiley & Sons Inc., with permission.)

Irradiate	^{1}H						^{19}F		
Observe	^{1}H	^{13}C	^{15}N	^{19}F	^{29}Si	^{31}P	^{1}H	^{13}C	^{19}F
η_{max}	0.5	1.99	−4.93	0.53	−2.52	1.24	0.47	1.87	0.5
$1 + \eta_{max}$	1.5	2.99	−3.93	1.53	−1.52	2.24	1.47	2.87	1.5

reasons for this. The nuclei may be directly bonded but the relaxation rate may be determined by mechanisms other than their direct through space interaction, such as an interaction with the solvent nuclei or paramagnetic impurities and we can then only observe a fraction of the possible η_{max}. This allows us to measure what proportion of the relaxation observed is due to the dipole–dipole mechanism since:

$$T_{1obs}/T_{1DD} = \eta_{obs}/\eta_{max}$$

Nuclear Overhauser studies thus allow us to investigate relaxation mechanisms. If quadrupolar relaxation is possible ($I > \frac{1}{2}$) then no Overhuaser effect is observed except in one or two very exceptional cases. η may also be reduced if the nuclei are not directly bonded so that they are further apart in space and if we can compare the values of η_{obs} for different nuclei S, S' in a molecule when a third spin I is irradiated then we can obtain a value for the ratio of distances $r_{IS}/r_{IS'}$. We have to be very careful in such measurements to ensure that only the dipole–dipole relaxation mechanism is present. Where the nucleus observed has a negative magnetogyric ratio it is possible for η_{obs} to have a value close to −1 when the total intensity will be close to zero. This is a real problem in ^{15}N and ^{29}Si spectroscopy where it may be necessary to suppress the Overhauser effect in some way. For positive magnetogyric ratio, and here we can think specifically of ^{13}C spectroscopy with proton broad band irradiation, a real increase in intensity for those carbon atoms directly bonded to hydrogen is obtained, whereas quaternary carbons show essentially no effect. Fig. 7.11 shows two spectra obtained with the same number of transients and other spectrometer settings but with and without broad band irradiation. The dramatic reduction in noise level is immediately apparent. The saving in

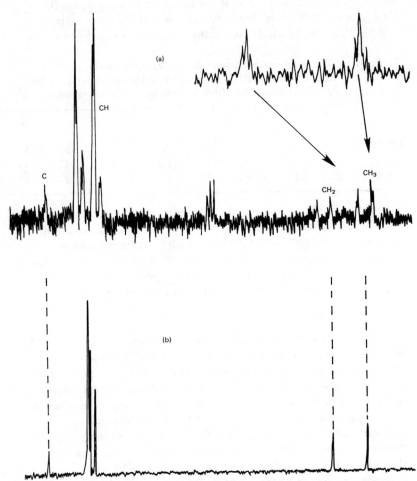

Figure 7.11   Carbon-13 spectra of ethyl benzene (a) non-decoupled
and (b) broad band decoupled. The decoupled spectrum is placed under
the non-decoupled spectrum so as to aid the positioning of the multiplets
of the latter. The improved signal to noise ratio in (b) arises because of
NOE effects and the removal of both long and short range spin—spin
couplings. The $CDCl_3$ solvent triplet is visible in (a) but not in (b)
because it lacks any NOE and so is very much smaller than the solute
resonances when these are decoupled. Only the central two lines of the
ethyl quartet are visible and these are split into triplets by the two bond
coupling to the methylene protons (inset, expanded horizontally). The
quaternary carbon is intensified in (b) to a smaller extent than the
others because it is further removed in space from any protons.

time is even more remarkable for it would require about 250 times as many accumulations to obtain the same signal to noise ratio for the methylene protons in the non-decoupled spectrum as is seen in the decoupled one. The intensities in these spectra are obviously very distorted and quantitative data is not available; we rely on the fact that carbon atoms are present in integral number ratios, and also have to assume our compounds are pure. Distortions arise also from the fact that such spectra are obtained with rather fast pulsing form the ^{13}C relaxation times which further reduces the intensity of the quaternary carbon resonances. There is obviously a wealth of information to be gained about these systems if we measure such factors as Overhauser enhancements, relaxation times, coupling patterns and natural intensity patterns. Accordingly, a variety of techniques have been devised, all based on pulse sequences.

Perhaps the simplest technique is however a chemical one in which chromium *tris*-acetylacetonate is added to the sample. This is a paramagnetic substance and its strong fluctuating magnetic field provides an alternative relaxation mechanism for the nuclei in the sample. ^{13}C relaxation times are much reduced and the nuclear Overhauser effect (abbreviated NOE) is suppressed. The method is good for rendering visible quaternary carbon atoms with very long relaxation times, but does involve contaminating the sample.

The instrumental techniques rely upon the fact that the NOE is determined by relaxation phenomena and takes times of the order of T_1 to become fully established whereas decoupling is established very quickly, within a few milliseconds. We can then devise sequences to obtain:

7.2.1 Full decoupling without NOE

This is achieved by decoupling only for the short time needed to collect the FID and then waiting sufficient time to allow any small NOE population changes to return to normal. The short pulse of B_2 does not allow appreciable build up of the NOE (Fig. 7.12).

7.2.2 No decoupling but full NOE

Here the decoupling power is left on for sufficient time for the NOE to build up to its full value and then switched off while the FID is collected (Fig. 7.13). This technique allows normal spectra to be obtained more quickly. If bad overlap to the multiplets occurs, an off resonance spectrum may be needed but normally it is possible to

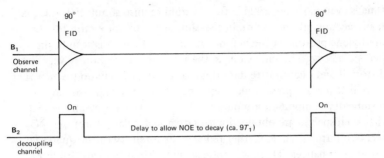

Figure 7.12   Decoupler timing to allow a fully decoupled spectrum to be obtained without any distortion of intensity due to the NOE. There will be a small build up of NOE during the B_2 pulse (typically $\frac{1}{2}$ s) and this must be allowed to die away completely before the next pulse. The long delay time means also that the nuclear magnetization has decayed fully before the next 90° pulse and there are no intensity distortions due to relaxation effects.

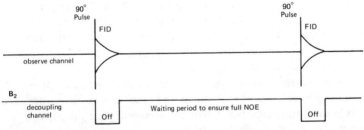

Figure 7.13   Decoupler timing to allow a non-decoupled spectrum to be obtained but with the benefit of the full NOE increase in intensities. There will be very little fall off in NOE during the short time needed to collect the FID data. This technique allows up to nine times reduction in time over the basic method used to obtain a non-decoupled spectrum.

distinguish quartets, triplets, doublets and singlets by a comparison with the decoupled spectrum and so to assign resonances to CH_3, CH_2, CH and quaternary carbons. It is well worth taking the trouble to carry out this experiment because the NOE enhancement can be about three times overall.

7.2.3   Measuring NOE and T_1

This is done by an experiment which is a combination of the two previous methods. The NOE is allowed to build up for a time t prior to producing the FID and this is collected while irradiation continues. B_2 is then switched off, the system allowed to equilibrate, and the process repeated. A series of experiments are run with different values of t (Fig. 7.14). Such experiments are known as dynamic NOE measurements and give both the Overhauser enhancement for each nucleus, and the value of T_1 from a suitable plot of the rate at which the NOE builds up with time. A dynamic NOE experiment with biphenyl is shown in Fig. 7.15 and the results are given in Table 7.2. Note the long relaxation time of the quaternary carbon and the fact that it has an NOE due to the long range interaction with the protons in the molecule ($\eta = (I_\infty/I_0) - 1$).

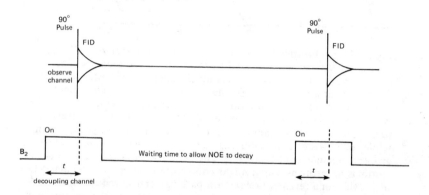

Figure 7.14   The dynamic NOE experiment. This is essentially a combination of the two experiments described by Figs 7.12 and 7.13. The decoupler is first gated On for a time t to allow the NOE to build up. The amount of NOE increases if t is increased, reaching a maximum when $t > 9T_1$. At the end of time t the FID is produced by the 90° pulse and collected with continuing irradiation. This is removed when the data collection is finished and the NOE allowed to decay to zero. Sufficient FIDs are collected to give the required signal to noise ratio and the experiment is repeated with different values of t, but always the same number of FIDs are collected so that spectral intensities can be compared directly. The results of a typical experiment are shown in Fig. 7.15.

This family of experiments is usually referred to as *gated decoupling* experiments. They are more time consuming than the simple population inversion technique described in Chapter 4, but give more detailed information about the interactions present in solutions.

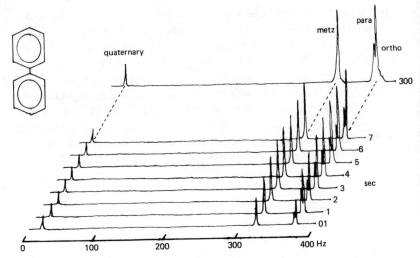

Figure 7.15   Fourier transform ^{13}C spectra of biphenyl in $CDCl_3$ excited by $90°$ pulses separated by intervals of 300 seconds. The assignment is based on the undecoupled spectrum. In order to illustrate the exponential build-up of the nuclear Overhauser enhancement, spectra are plotted as a function of t, the period for which the protons were preirradiated with a noise decoupler before the ^{13}C excitation pulse. These time constants give the ^{13}C spin–lattice relaxation times, while the ratios of corresponding intensities in the first and last spectra give the enhancement factors η. The solvent $CDCl_3$ is used because it contains no protons which might contribute to an intermolecular NOE or provide an alternative relaxation pathway and so reduce the intramolecular NOE. The small magnetic moments of the deuteron and chlorine will have little effect on relaxation rates of the solute, though it is of course essential to ensure that dissolved paramagnetic oxygen is absent. (Reproduced with permission from Freeman, Hill and Kaptein (1972) *J. Mag. Res.*, **7**, 327.)

Table 7.2   *Experimental spin–lattice relaxation times and nuclear Overhauser enhancement factors for ^{13}C nuclei in biphenyl*

Carbon nucleus	T_1 (seconds)	I_∞/I_0
Quaternary	54 ± 4	2.00 ± 0.16
Meta	5.4 ± 0.7	2.80 ± 0.21
Para	3.4 ± 0.6	2.72 ± 0.16
Ortho	5.2 ± 0.8	2.76 ± 0.19

7.3   Selective population inversion

The experiments outlined in Section 7.2 rely on changes introduced in
the nuclear populations of the various energy levels when one is
irradiated and they are coupled via the relaxation pathways. Pulse
techniques, however, allow us to change spin populations drastically
and controllably simply by subjecting the nuclei to an inverting 180°
pulse. The resulting return to equilibrium is accompanied by significant,
and in some cases, very large, changes in intensity of the lines due to
coupled transitions, magnified if the magnetogyric ratio of the inverted
spin is greater than that of the observed spin. The method is particularly
useful for assisting in the observation of quaternary carbon atoms with
long relaxation times, since the effective relaxation time in such an
experiment is that of the inverted proton and this is usually much
shorter than that of the carbon. An example is given in Fig. 7.16 for
the carbonyl carbon of acetone. The proton spectrum of acetone
contains two sets of ^{13}C satellites, one pair widely spaced and due to
coupling to directly bonded ^{13}C in the methyl groups, and one with a
much smaller coupling constant due to the two bond coupling between
the methyl protons and the carbonyl ^{13}C. The carbonyl ^{13}C resonance
is therefore split into a septet with line intensities 1:6:15:20:15:6:1 by
this coupling. If we invert the proton spins corresponding to one of the
inner ^{13}C satellites by irradiating this with a long, selective 180° pulse
and follow this immediately with a pulse at the ^{13}C frequency to
stimulate a ^{13}C FID we find that the carbonyl carbon intensities have
been greatly perturbed and now have the intensities +25:+102:+135:
+20:−105:−90:−23, which is a useful gain in intensity.

7.4   Double resonance and exchange coupling

We have already seen that slow exchange of atoms between two sites A
and B leads to line broadening. The areas of the lines of the exchanging
nuclei however remain constant since the populations of the high and
low energy states remain unperturbed as the same proportion of nuclei
arrive at or leave each type of site in the low energy state. If though we
were to alter the population ratio at site A by irradiating the resonance
at its nuclear frequency then this perturbation would arrive at site B
and its rate of appearance would allow conclusions to be drawn about
the rate of exchange. An example is given in Fig. 7.17. Here we measure
the magnetization of a given carbon atom while a chemically shifted

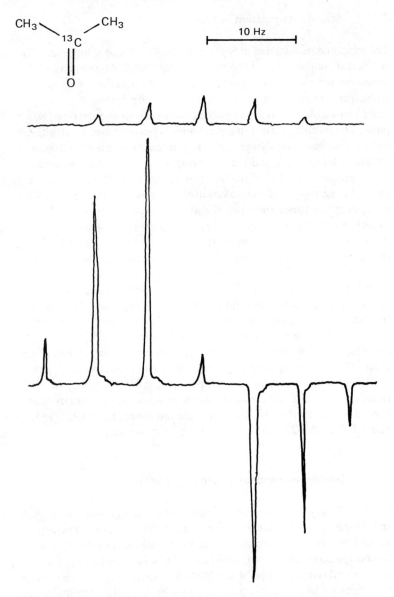

Figure 7.16 A heteronuclear selective population inversion experiment. The ^{13}C spectrum of the carbonyl group of acetone is a septet due to coupling to the protons of the two methyl groups. If a 180° selective pulse is applied at the proton frequency of one of the carbonyl ^{13}C satellites (the high field one in this case) and then the

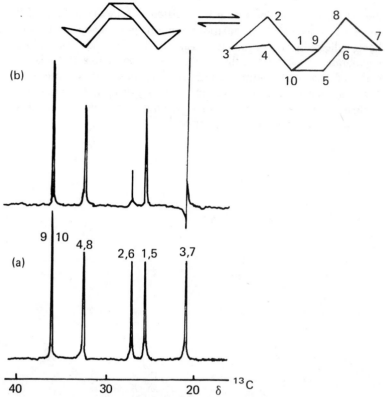

(b)

9 | 10   4,8   2,6   1,5   3,7

(a)

40   30   20 δ ^{13}C

Figure 7.17   An FT measurement of the rate of slow interchange of the carbon positions in *cis*-decalin as the rings flex. Irradiation of the 3,7 carbon resonance reduces the intensity of the 2,6 carbon resonance in (b) over that in the non-irradiated spectrum (a). The solvent is CD_2Cl_2 and temperature 226 K. The relaxation time is measured in a separate experiment and the average residence time in a site is then given by

$$\tau = [M_z(\infty)/\{M_z(0) - M_z(\infty)\}]T_1$$

where $M_z(0)$ is the line intensity without irradiation of the other and $M_z(\infty)$ is that after irradiation has been applied sufficiently long for equilibrium to have been obtained, ca. T_1 s. (After Mann (1976) *J. Mag. Res.*, **21**, 17 with permission.)

---

^{13}C FID stimulated, large enhancements of all the line intensities in the carbon spectrum are obtained. This is particularly obvious for the outer lines of the normal, undecoupled spectrum (upper trace) which are not visible in the noise but have become high intensity lines after the inversion. The value of $^2J(CH)$ is 5.92 Hz. (After Jakobsen, Linde and Sorensen (1974) *J. Mag. Res.*, **15**, 385 with permission.)

one which is exchanging with it is irradiated. A time shared method has to be used since the ^{13}C irradiation cannot be present while data is being collected so that irradiation is applied for a period sufficient to equilibrate the system and then the nuclear response to a 90° pulse collected. The equilibrium magnetization depends upon the rate of exchange and the rate of relaxation, the two arriving at a balance. The exchange rate can therefore be calculated if T_1 is known, and this has to be measured in a separate experiment.

8

Some New and Exciting Techniques in NMR

We intend to deal here with a number of topics which are recent and which would not normally be considered appropriate for a text book at this level. We do however seem to be witnessing at the moment another surge in the development of NMR spectroscopy which promises to be at least as productive as that which occurred when FT spectroscopy was introduced. This time though the developments are taking place on several fronts and are contributing to quite different areas, even to the extent that we may stray a little from what is purely chemistry, though all the techniques are bound by the fact that they rely on pulsed NMR and the existence of the minicomputer. These then are all worth knowing about and are presented in no particular order.

8.1   Two-dimensional NMR

The spectra so far described are one dimensional in the sense that the FID we obtain is a function of a single time variable. It is possible to introduce a second time variable by subjecting the spins to some treatment for a time τ which can be varied, prior to collecting the FID in the normal way. The FID will then have a form which depends upon the treatment and upon τ. We can then collect a series of FIDs corresponding to different values of τ and obtain spectra via a two-dimensional Fourier transform to give a plot of intensities spread over a two-dimensional field in a way which can be predetermined by the manipulations of the data. One way in which this can be done is shown in Fig. 8.1. The pulse sequence used is one which will produce a spin echo (p. 92 and Fig. 4.18). The spins are subjected to a 90° pulse and the resulting output ignored. After a certain time interval, which can be

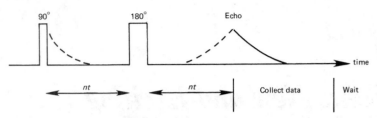

Figure 8.1   The spin echo sequence as used to obtain proton two-dimensional *J* spectra. The 90° pulse gives an FID. After some time *nt*, where *n* can have a series of values, 1,2,3, . . . , a 180° pulse is applied to refocus the spins. This is followed by a spin echo which reaches a maximum at time *nt* after this second pulse, at which point data collection is started. A series of FIDs are obtained for many different *n* and then subjected to a two-dimensional Fourier transform. Note that the pulsewidths are much exaggerated in this type of diagram.

varied in steps, a 180° refocusing pulse is applied and the nuclear magnetization builds up again to reach a maximum at double the chosen time interval and data collection is then started. The sequence can be repeated after a suitable delay to allow equilibriation so as to enhance the signal to noise ratio. The experiment is then repeated with the time interval incremented. The resulting family of FIDs contain components at the frequency of each line in the spectrum but each with different phase relationships, depending on τ. A plot of transformed FIDs obtained in this way from a solution of trideuteriomethyl 2,3,4,6-tetrakis-O-trideuterioacetyl-α-D-glucopyranoside is shown in Fig. 8.2. A series of plots are obtained which are displayed side by side. All the lines which originate from a proton of a particular chemical shift appear at that shift position but spread out on the other frequency axis to show their full multiplicity. The refocusing feature of the experiment means that the resolution is very good so that, for instance, H4, which is a triplet in the normal spectrum, is shown to be a doublet of doublets. The projection of these spectra on the shift axis gives a series of singlets which is in fact the normally unattainable *broad band homonuclear* double irradiation spectrum. The new information in this spectrum in this example is not large, especially when it is realized that two hours are required for the experiment. The power of the method is however, shown in Fig. 8.3 for the larger molecule cellobiose where the normal spectrum shows extensive overlap. In such a complex case it is very difficult to be sure of the assignments of the proton resonances. A variety of double resonance difference spectra using decoupling or

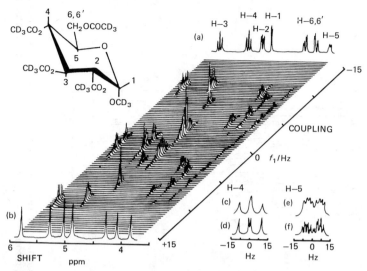

Figure 8.2   270 MHz proton spectra of a deuteriated glucopyranoside.
(a) shows the normal spectrum and its assignment, placed parallel with
the δ scale. (b) the chemical shift projection with all coupling lost. The
coupling patterns can be seen by following the changes in intensity
which occur parallel to the f_1 axis. The inset spectra (c), (d) and (e),
(f) compare the normal multiplet (upper) with the 2D multiplet (lower).
The spectra were taken on a 0.1 M solution in deuterio benzene. Note
that the pair of methylene protons 6,6′ give an AB quartet showing
further small couplings. (Reproduced with permission from Hall,
Sukuma and Sullivan (1979) *J. Chem. Soc. Chem. Commun.*, 292.)

NOE effects may help and useful information can be obtained by
correlating the proton lines with the ^{13}C spectrum, since the ^{13}C shifts
are much more widely dispersed and can be assigned relatively straightforwardly for such molecules. This can also be achieved in a single step
using a two-dimensional technique which obtains the ^{13}C spectrum
normally but introduces timing into the commencement of the proton
broad band irradiation so as to obtain the other dimension relating the
two different nuclear species. The experiment is started with a 90° pulse
at the ^{13}C frequency and in the absence of broad band irradiation of
^1H. This produces ^{13}C magnetization which commences to precess in
the xy plane. We do not collect data. The carbon resonances will each
have a particular frequency and multiplicity, and if we think of say a
doublet, each component will have a different angular frequency and
the corresponding nuclei will have different orientations in space after

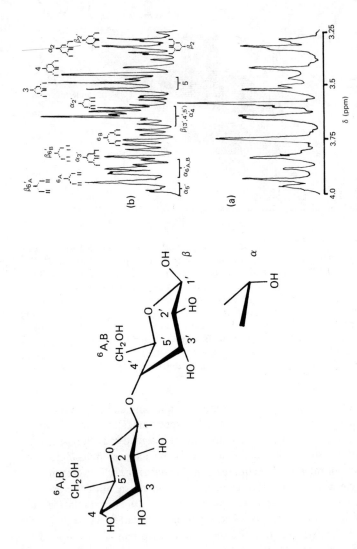

Figure 8.3   270 MHz proton spectra of cellobiose. The upper is the normal spectrum and the lower is the two-dimensional J spectrum with all the homonuclear couplings removed (nonanomeric resonances) and therefore containing only chemical shift information. (Reproduced with permission from Hall, Morris and Sukuma (1980) *J. Amer. Chem. Soc.*, **102**, 1745.)

some time τ. We then switch on the decoupler and the two components then precess at the same frequency but each with a different phase so that their combined intensity is a function of τ. The collection of the FID is started at the same time as the decoupler. Sufficient responses are accumulated to give an adequate signal to noise ratio and then the experiment is repeated with a different τ to give the required series of FIDs ready for two-dimensional transformation. The two-dimensional plot thus contains corresponding proton and carbon-13 data. A fuller discussion of the possibilities will be found in the *Journal of the American Chemical Society* (1980) **102**, p. 5703, relating to the spectra of 1-dehydrotestosterone. Many pulse sequences have now been developed for this type of work and to probe different facets of spin systems, and can for instance allow forbidden and multi quantum transitions to be observed.

8.2   Whole body imaging

This is a very important new technique of application to the medical field which allows us access to body chemistry, hence its inclusion here. Its commercial importance can be judged from the fact that three groups are involved in its development separately in the UK, and others elsewhere, particularly the USA. It relies upon the fact that within the body there are concentrations of mobile protons which can give an NMR resonance and whose concentration varies depending upon the type of tissue observed. The apparatus used for such observation is completely different from that so far encountered here. The magnet is a physically large, low magnetic field device with a sample gap sufficiently large to take an adult person. A large air filled solenoid is used. The magnetic field has impressed upon it magnetic field gradients which can be manipulated so as to define a sensitive spot within the sample where the protons are in resonance. The sensitive spot can be moved around and the proton density mapped over a section of the subject. There is some evidence that cancerous tissue has a different relaxation time to that of normal tissue and this sort of change can also be mapped. Ways of speeding up the data collection are being worked out and a pulse sequence which can give a series of responses from a sensitive plane can currently give an image in a few seconds. A great deal of computing power is of course needed to achieve this end, and resolutions of the order of 2 to 3 mm are obtainable. The method should be complementary to that of X-ray scanning since it picks signals up from the softer body tissues, and indeed operates without any apparent hazard to the subject. NMR spectroscopists can rest assured that it seems their technique is non-hazardous. The technique is also described as zeugmatography or tomography.

8.3   *In vivo* biological investigations

In addition to the mobile protons in a living organism, there are molecules containing ^{13}C and ^{31}P nuclei which can also be used for study of how the chemistry of life operates. Early experiments with whole, anaesthetized, small animals in large bore magnets were promising but signals were obtained from all parts of the animal. It quickly became clear that it would be of most use if signals could be localized to a specific known organ. One approach is to create a specially contoured magnetic field which has the correct value for resonance over only a small, controllable volume. It is possible, for instance, to follow the ^{31}P signals of nucleotide phosphates and inorganic phosphate in muscle and monitor how these respond to different conditions imposed on the muscle. An example of 'topical NMR' as it is called, is given in Fig. 8.4 which demonstrates the effect on the ^{31}P spectrum of a subject's arm of applying a tourniquet. These techniques are showing promise as an aid in kidney transplant surgery where it is possible to monitor the viability of a donor organ prior to transplant, and, in principle, to monitor its behaviour after insertion in the recipient.

Other biological studies involve rather heterogenious samples which the NMR spectroscopist would rather tend to avoid. The advent of the high field spectrometers has, however, meant that worse resolution can be accepted and results are now being reported for samples such as cell suspensions or living perfused organs. A ^{31}P spectrum of perfused rat liver is shown in Fig. 8.6 and is of interest because two sorts of inorganic phosphate are visible, inside and outside the cells. This arises because there is a pH difference between the two regions and there is a pH dependent shift of ^{31}P due to the protonation reaction

$$H_2PO_4^- \rightleftharpoons HPO_4^{2-}$$

The chemical shift is a weighted average of the shifts of the two ions (0.4 and 3.0 ppm) which undergo rapid exchange, and whose relative populations vary with pH. Metabolic pathways can be followed in similar samples using ^{13}C spectroscopy if ^{13}C enriched substrates are added to the sample. Fig. 8.7 shows the spectrum obtained by

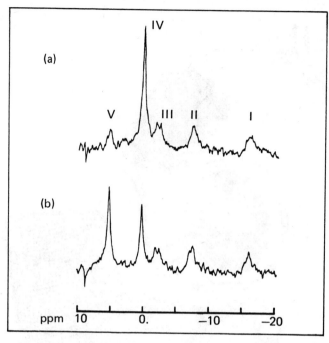

Figure 8.4 ^{31}P topical NMR spectra obtained at 32.5 MHz using a single turn coil placed on the surface of the subject's arm, in a contoured magnetic field. (a) shows the spectrum obtained from 64 two second scans from human forearm muscle. The peaks I, II and III arise from the three phosphorus atoms in adenosine triphosphate (ATP), IV from phosphocreatine and V from inorganic phosphate. Other minor phosphorus containing components are also present but are not resolved. (b) is the same subject 50 minutes after the application of a tourniquet to the upper arm and shows how oxygen starvation leads to breakdown of the organic phosphates to inorganic phosphate. (Reproduced with permission from Gordon (1981) *Europ. Spect. News*, 38, 21.)

accumulating data between the 18th and 35th minutes after adding 1,3-^{13}C-glycerol to rat liver cells. The ^{13}C label appears in the 1,3,4 and 6 carbons of glucose and peaks due to L-glyceryl 3-phosphate are also visible. Certain of the glucose carbons show carbon–carbon spin coupling since enrichment leads to there being more than one ^{13}C atom in each molecule. Another way in which such enrichment spectra can be obtained is to run two proton spectra, one with and one without ^{13}C

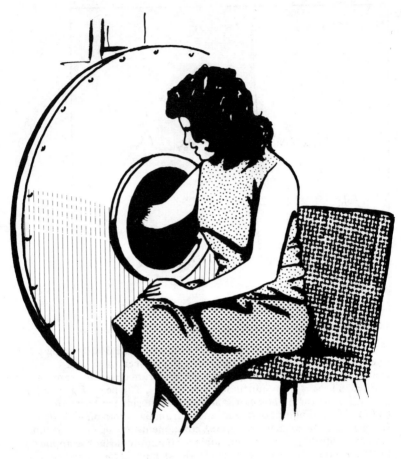

Figure 8.5   A human NMR sample. (Reproduced with permission from *European Spectroscopy News* (1981) **38**, front cover.)

double irradiation and take the difference. This removes all the background and unaffected resonances and leaves only those coupled to ^{13}C enriched carbon locations.

8.4   High resolution solid state NMR

Chemists have only had a limited interest in solid state NMR because the resonances are very broad, often of the order of 50 kHz, and all the structure so useful in high resolution work is lost. Because the line-width

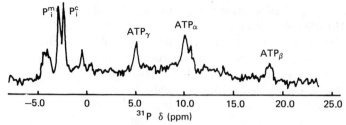

Figure 8.6 ^{31}P NMR spectrum of perfused rat liver cells. The two inorganic phosphate peaks P_i arise from phosphate in the mitochondria and cytosol, the latter being sensitive to the external pH while the former changes very little. The three lines marked ATP are from the three phosphorus atoms in adenosine triphosphate. The pH difference has been increased by adding valinomycin which is an ionophore for K^+. (Reproduced with permission from Shulman *et al.* (1979) *Science*, **205**, 160.)

is a function of the internuclear distance it has been possible in simple cases to measure proton–proton distances, which is of use since they are difficult to obtain by other means. The line shape also depends upon the number of spins in an interacting cluster and in many crystalline hydrates it is possible to distinguish whether the water of crystallisation is present as H_2O, H_3O^+ or OH^-. For instance borax $Na_2O \cdot 2B_2O_3 \cdot 10H_2O$ has been shown to have the structure $Na_2[B_4O_5(OH)_4]$ $8H_2O$, a hydrated scandium nitrate, $Sc_4O_3(NO_3)_6 \cdot 7H_2O$ should be formulated $[Sc_4O(OH)_4](NO_3)_6 \cdot 5H_2O$, while a hydrated form of gallium sulphate contains both hydronium ion and hydroxide ions and is $(H_3O)Ga_3(OH)_6(SO_4)_2$.

If the interacting spins are moving so that their relative orientations change. e.g. by rotation of the group of atoms around some axis, then their through space coupling and the line-width of their resonance is reduced. Thus by measuring line-widths at a series of temperatures, information can be obtained about the state of motion of various groups in a crystal. Fig. 8.8 shows the line-widths of the solid state proton spectra obtained from the complex adduct of trimethylamine and boron trifluoride, $(CH_3)_3N{\rightarrow}BF_3$. At 68 K there is no rotation around the CN bonds and the line is at its broadest. As the temperature is increased to 103 K a marked narrowing occurs which marks the onset of rotation of the methyl groups around the CN bond. Further narrowing occurs between 100 K and 150 K and this is due to the onset of rotation of the whole $N(CH_3)_3$ molecule around the B–N bond. Finally just below 400 K the line narrows to a fraction of a gauss as the whole molecule starts to rotate isotropically and to diffuse within the still *solid* crystal.

The fluorine resonance of the BF_3 part of the molecule is broad only below 77 K and the BF_3 group rotates around the B–N axis at all higher temperatures. Changes in the line-widths can often be associated with phase transitions observed by other means.

This example does not of course comprise high resolution work. What we ideally wish to achieve in the solid state is the same sort of spectrum that we obtain from a solution of the substance; without the dipolar line broadening. The realization of such an ideal would open up whole new areas of study of solid substances. It has consequently received much attention, and three lines of attack have developed and are now coming together in commercially realizable form; magic angle spinning, high power double irradiation, and pulse techniques.

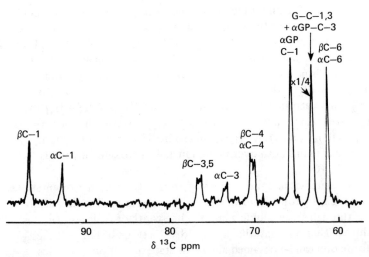

Figure 8.7   Carbon-13 NMR spectrum at $25°C$ of rat liver cells from a normal rat, accumulated between 18 and 35 minutes after the introduction of 22 mM $[1,3\text{-}^{13}C]$ glycerol. Glucose is labelled strongly at the 1, 3, 4, and 6 carbon positions of the α and β anomers of glucose. Note that the carbon-carbon spin coupling has split the lines from C-3 and C-4 of glucose. G-C-1,3 is the labelled glycerol peak, and αGP is L-glycerol 3-phosphate. The carbon–carbon coupling splits the glucose resonances apparently into triplets because these are superpositions of the singlet due to the molecules containing only one ^{13}C between the lines of the doublet due to those containing two ^{13}C atoms. (Reproduced with permission from Shulman *et al.* (1979) *Science*, **205**, 160.)

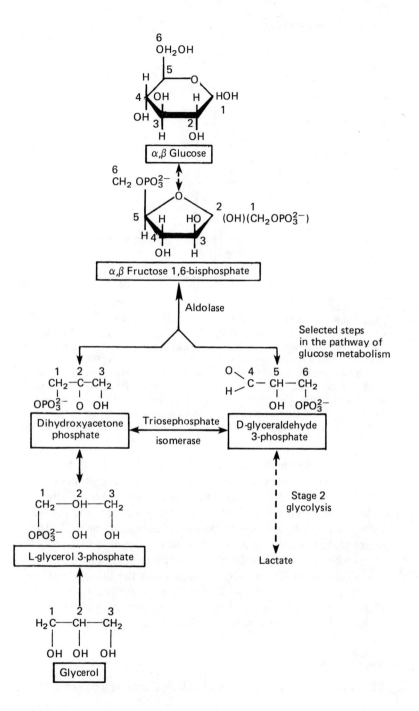

Selected steps in the pathway of glucose metabolism

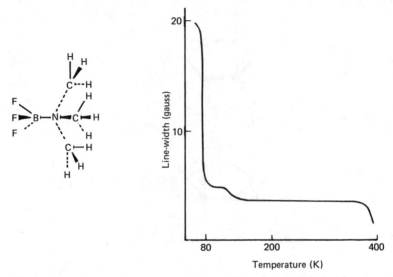

Figure 8.8   The proton resonance line-width of the methylamine protons in the solid adduct $(CH_3)_3 N \rightarrow BF_3$ as a function of temperature. The spectra were developed by sweeping the field, 1 gauss being equivalent to a frequency interval in this case of 4250 Hz. The line-width thus varies from about 85 kHz to 13 kHz while the sample is cool and solid and falls further as extensive internal diffusion occurs near the melting point. Finally of course, the line-width falls to a fraction of a Hz (say 1/200 000 of the scale shown) when the sample melts. (After Dunnel, *et al.* (1969) *Trans. Faraday Soc.*, **65**, 1153, with permission.)

There are three problems of solid samples which have to be overcome: (1) the lines are broadened due to the through space interactions of the spins which have to be reduced to zero. If the nucleus observed has a quadrupole moment this gives rise to further broadening by interaction with electric fields in the sample. (2) The chemical shift anisotropy shows up in the absence of motion so that if the molecules take several directions relative to the magnetic field (they take all directions for a powdered sample) then the chemical shift anisotropy adds to the line-width. (3) T_1 is extremely long in solids. This limits the rate at which data can be acquired and has to be overcome in some way if we are to observe the less receptive spin $\frac{1}{2}$ nuclei.

8.4.1   Magic angle spinning

The magnetic field produced by a nucleus, magnetic moment μ, at a second nucleus a distance r away is, in the z or $\mathbf{B_0}$ direction, given by:

$$H_b = (K \, \mu/r^3)(3 \cos^2\theta - 1)$$

where K is a constant and θ is the angle between the $\mathbf{B_0}$ field direction and the line joining the two nuclei. When this is at an angle of 54°44′ to the field, the value of H_b is zero and the nuclei cannot perturb $\mathbf{B_0}$ at each others locations, and so cannot affect their resonant frequencies (Fig. 8.9). In fact all values of θ will be found in a typical solid sample. If we mount the sample as a cylinder with its axis at an angle of 54°44′ to the main field direction and spin it rapidly around this axis, each internuclear vector will gain an average value which lies at 54°44′ to the field, its average H_b will be zero, and all broadening should disappear. Thus the angle 54°44′ is known as the magic angle. The quadrupole interaction and chemical shift anisotropies also follow $3\cos^2\theta - 1$ laws and they too are eliminated by magic angle spinning (Fig. 8.10 and 8.11). The main limitation to the method is the speed of rotation which should be greater in Hz than the line-width. Technical

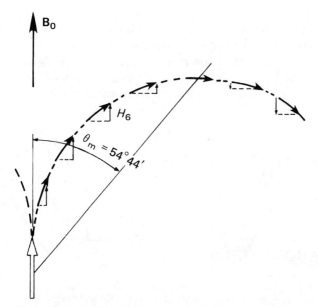

Figure 8.9   A line of the magnetic field originating from a magnetic dipole has zero z component at a point situated on a line originating at the centre of the dipole and at an angle of 54°44′ to the direction of the dipole. (From Bruker CXP application notes.)

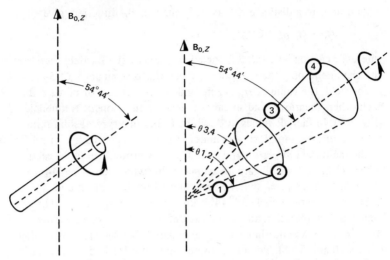

Figure 8.10   Showing how a solid sample is mounted for magic angle spinning and how this gives the internuclear vectors an average orientation at the spinning angle. (From Bruker CXP application notes.)

requirements limit this to about 7 kHz. Thus we would not expect to remove all effects of directly bonded protons which give the maximum line-widths. We are aided in the adamantane spectrum shown in Fig. 8.11 by the fact there is also molecular motion in the solid, since this sphere-like molecule can rotate easily and the interactions are then reduced.

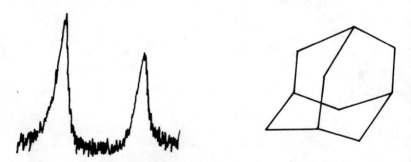

Figure 8.11   The ^{13}C spectrum of adamantane in the solid state, with magic angle spinning. The resonances are about 200 Hz wide whereas in the static solid the dipole—dipole interactions with the protons increase the linewidth to approaching 5000 Hz and the individual chemical shifts are not resolved. (Spectrum from Bruker CXP application notes.)

Obviously, further improvements are needed to this basic technique, though Fig. 8.12 shows that marked improvements can be obtained in ^{31}P NMR and good results have also been reported for ^{23}Na and ^{27}Al. It is nevertheless already finding use in examining the aromatic/aliphatic ratio in coal samples.

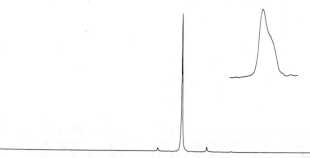

Figure 8.12 ^{31}P spectra of ammonium dihydrogen phosphate, $(NH_4)H_2PO_4$, in the solid state, with and without magic angle spinning. The resonance from the non-spinning sample shows the typical shape of a line broadened by chemical shift anisotropy. Spinning reduces the line-width by a factor of 24 times. Note the spinning sidebands, which can be a nuisance in complex spectra. The non-spinning line-width is 6800 Hz. (From Bruker CXP application notes.)

8.4.2   *Dilute isotopes with high power double resonance*

Here we will consider specifically solid state ^{13}C spectra. The ^{13}C nuclei are only 1.1% abundant and so will not be situated close to one another. Line broadening will thus be caused mainly by the protons and, to a lesser extent, other abundant nuclei such as ^{14}N if present in the molecules. The effect of the protons can be much reduced by irradiating them strongly at their resonant frequency which will cause them to precess around B_2 and so appear to have an average zero magnetic moment. Again, the effectiveness of the method is limited by the requirement that sufficient power must be provided to cover the whole proton line-width, which requires transmitters of 100 W feeding power into rather restricted spaces. Fig. 8.13 shows what can be done with adamantane using this technique and Fig. 8.14 demonstrates the very real improvement obtained by combining double resonance with magic angle spinning.

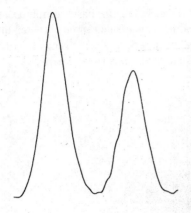

Figure 8.13   The ^{13}C spectrum of adamantane in the solid state, with high power decoupling of the protons with a power equivalent to 48 kHz. Here the lines are about 450 Hz wide. (From Bruker CXP application notes.)

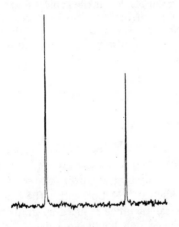

Figure 8.14   The ^{13}C spectrum of adamantane with both magic angle spinning and double irradiation. The line-width is now 2 Hz. (From Bruker CXP application notes.)

8.4.3   Cross polarization in conjunction with the above

It remains to overcome the problems associated with the extended relaxation times of nuclei in solid samples. This is done by causing an energy flow from the few ^{13}C nuclei towards the numerous ^{1}H nuclei, which act as a nuclear heat sink, and so increase the population of the low energy ^{13}C spin state. This increases the intensity of the ^{13}C signal and also provides an extra relaxation pathway. In order that energy exchange shall be possible between the two nuclear species we must introduce components of motion with the same frequency for each. This is done as follows. Referring to Fig. 8.15, we first prepare the protons for the cross polarization by applying a short $90°$ pulse which swings the protons into the xy plane. We will call this field $\mathbf{B}_{1H}$. We then simultaneously reduce $\mathbf{B}_{1H}$ and change its phase by $90°$ so that

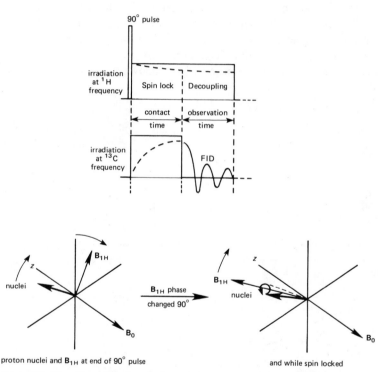

Figure 8.15   Showing the timing of the various events in a cross polarization experiment. A $90°$ pulse at the proton frequency is followed by a long spin locking pulse changed in phase from the initial pulse by $90°$ which prevents the normal proton relaxation processes. Energy is caused to flow from the assembly of ^{13}C nuclei to the cooled proton nuclei by applying a long pulse at the ^{13}C frequency which introduces a precession frequency equal to that already established for the protons. When equilibrium is reached, this field is switched off and is followed by a ^{13}C FID of enhanced intensity.

the B_{1H} vector becomes parallel with the spins in the xy plane. The spins remain in the xy plane and stay there locked to B_{1H}, which is known as a spin locking pulse. The magnetization of the spin vector cone precesses in the xy plane at the Larmor frequency and the distribution in the cone can be thought of as also precessing around B_{1H} at a frequency of $\gamma_H B_{1H}/2\pi$ Hz, behaving as if they were very strongly polarized in the weak B_{1H}. Reference to Equation 1.1 will show that such a polarization, correct under normal circumstances for B_0, can only be attained if the temperature is very low for a field B_{1H}, and we can consider that the spin locking has cooled the spins which can now act as an energy sink. Energy transfer is obtained by applying a long pulse at the ^{13}C frequency, B_{1C}, which has an amplitude such that the ^{13}C nuclei precess around B_0 at a frequency of $\gamma_C B_{1C}/2\pi$ which is equal to $\gamma_H B_{1H}/2\pi$. The identical frequency components allow energy transfer, which follows an exponential curve,

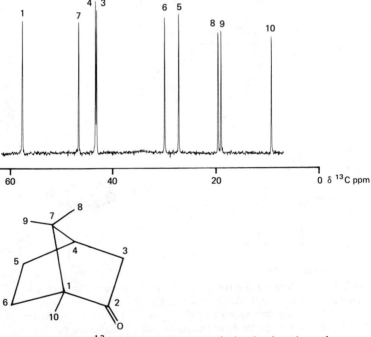

Figure 8.16   The ^{13}C, solid state, cross polarization/magic angle spinning spectrum (abbreviated CPMAS) of camphor. The spectrum is comparable with the liquid state spectrum. The assignments are given based on the liquid state. The CO carbon is not shown; its chemical shift is 216.7 ppm. (From Bruker CXP leaflet.)

and when this has reached a maximum the $\mathbf{B}_{1C}$ is cut off and is followed by a ^{13}C FID of enhanced intensity. The $\mathbf{B}_{1H}$ field remains on during this time and provides the decoupling of the protons from the carbon. Some idea of the sort of spectra which can be obtained is given in Fig. 8.16.

8.4.4   Pulse spinning

If the nuclei are not dilute then the magnetic interactions between them are large and the above methods will not give high resolution. We could for instance think of examining the protons in ice. In this case the magnetic interactions are eliminated by causing the spins themselves to swing about the magnetic field direction by applying a series of 90° pulses along both the x and y axes and by alternating their phases. The spins can be caused to move very quickly, much more rapidly than by a mechanical method, but the pulses have to be very short and of high power and separated by very short time intervals, so that the method is technically very difficult. Repetitive pulse trains have been designed using 4, 8, 24 and 52 pulses. The data is sampled during certain intervals in the pulse train and collected in memory. Some recent results for hexagonal ice at liquid nitrogen temperature are shown in Fig. 8.17. The unit cell is such that the eight different OH. . .O bonds have seven different directions in space. The chemical shift of each proton is therefore determined by different admixtures of the chemical shift with the field perpendicular to the bond and that with it parallel, i.e. by the chemical shift anisotropy and the position of the crystal in the magnetic field. Five lines can be resolved and these allow the chemical shift anisotropy to be calculated as $\sigma_{\parallel} = 16.0$ ppm and $\sigma_{\perp} = -12.5$ ppm relative to liquid water at room temperature.

8.5   High pressure NMR

Studies at high pressure are carried out in spectrometers which operate in standard ways except that the sample is contained in a high pressure bomb, together with the detection coil, and its pressure can be varied externally. Care has to be taken with construction and shimming since it is not possible to spin the sample. Experiments have been carried out with systems where the rates of exchange are dependent upon the pressure and the spectra obtained resemble those in variable temperature runs. The technique is particularly useful in that it allows us to measure

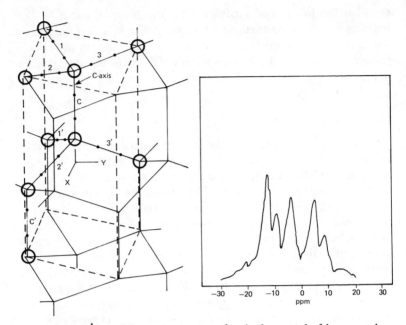

Figure 8.17 ^{1}H solid state spectrum of a single crystal of hexagonal ice at liquid nitrogen temperature obtained using a 52 pulse sequence. The diagram on the left shows the crystal structure with circles indicating the oxygen positions and dots the two possible hydrogen positions in each OH. . .O hydrogen bond. Only one of these positions can be occupied. (After Rhim, Burum and Elleman (1979) *J. Chem. Phys.*, **71**, 3139, with permission.)

volume changes which occur during chemical exchange reactions. Thus in the reaction

$$MX_5.L + L' \rightleftharpoons MX_5.L' + L \text{ (L = a ligand, X = halide, M = metal)}$$

the ligand exchange may proceed via the intermediate transition states MX_5 (dissociative exchange) or $MX_5.L_2$ (associative exchange). The overall volume of the first ($MX_5 + 2L$) will be larger than that of the initial reactants so that increased pressure would be expected slow down down the exchange, the converse being true for the second scheme. In the case of the dissociative mechanism the rate determining step leads to a first order rate law. If C is the concentration of the complex $MX_5.L$ then the reaction is

$$C \underset{k_{-1}}{\overset{k_1}{\rightleftharpoons}} MX_5 + L \qquad 1/\tau_c = -dC/Cdt = k_1$$

and τ_c is obtained by an analysis of the NMR line-shape. For the associative mechanism the rate determining step leads to a second order rate law.

$$C + L \xrightleftharpoons[k_{-2}]{k_2} CL \qquad 1/\tau_c = -dC/Cdt = k_2 \text{ [free L]}$$

k_1 or k_2 is determined as a function of pressure and the volume of activation obtained from a plot of $\ln k$ against pressure since

$$\Delta V^* = -RT(\delta \ln k/\delta P)_T$$

Two typical sets of results are depicted in Fig. 8.18, for the associative

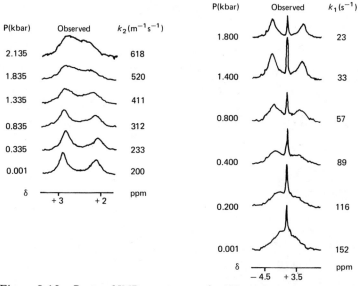

Figure 8.18   Proton NMR spectra as a function of pressure in systems undergoing exchange. On the left we are observing exchange of dimethyl sulphide on its complex with tantalum pentabromide, in the presence of excess sulphide. A doublet is observed due to $Me_2S.TaBr_5$ and free Me_2S at low pressure where exchange is therefore slow. Increased pressure causes the doublet to coalesce and so must increase the rate of exchange. It must thus increase the concentration of transition state which must then be of lower volume. The exchange is associative with a negative volume of activation. On the right we have the results for the system $Me_2O + TaBr_5.Me_2O$ where exchange is only slow enough to observe separate bound and free ether signals at high pressure. This exchange is therefore dissociative with a positive volume of activation. The sharp peak is a ^{13}C satellite of the solvent CH_2Cl_2. (After Merbach (1977) *Helv. Chim. Acta*, **60**, 1124 with permission.)

exchange of Me_2S on $TaBr_5$. Me_2S where the rate is increased by applying pressure and ΔV^* has the value -12.6 cm^3 mol^{-1}, and for the dissociative exchange of Me_2O on $TaBr_5.Me_2O$ where the rate is decreased by applying pressure and ΔV^* has the value $+30.5$ cm^3 mol^{-1}. The volume of activation, as might be expected, is not independent of pressure over the large ranges of pressure change discussed here and the ln k/P plots are curved. The ΔV^* values are then obtained by extrapolation to zero pressure using a quadratic fit to the experimental curve.

9
Some Examples of the Use of NMR in Chemistry

The object of this chapter is to indicate how the various principles outlined in the previous chapters are applied in practice. Some of the examples are presented as problems while the more complex ones are wholly or partly worked through.

An attempt has been made to cover as wide a variety of topics as is possible. This means unfortunately that no single topic can be given a very full treatment and particularly that the use of NMR by the preparative chemist for the determination of the structures of organic compounds is given a far smaller proportion of space than its use deserves. This is inevitable in a book of this size and the student is referred to the bibliography where he will find mention of several books which cover this aspect more fully.

Part A Proton and carbon spectroscopy

9.1 The determination of the structures of organic molecules using proton spectra

One example will be worked through and the remainder are left for the student to attempt to solve. The formulae of the substances giving the spectra are reproduced at the end of the section but are not assigned to individual spectra. That is left to the student.

Several complementary pieces of information can be obtained from an NMR spectrum and should be considered in turn when analysing a trace. First we have the chemical shift information and a guide to the meaning of this can be found from the simplified chart of Fig. 9.1.

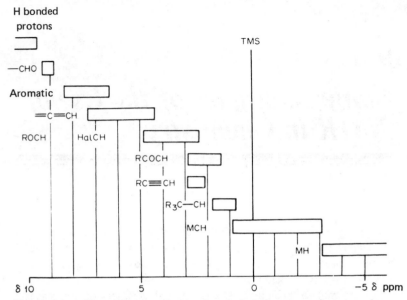

Figure 9.1   Chart of approximate chemical shift ranges of protons in organic and organo-metallic compounds. M represents a metal and Hal a halogen.

Secondly there is the spin coupling information which allows us to count numbers of proximate protons. Thirdly there is the intensity data which allows us to determine the relative numbers of each type of proton. This is not necessarily the same thing as is found from spin coupling data, since for instance a compound might contain one, two, or more identical ethyl groups. Intensities can sometimes be obtained by inspection, but because lines have different breadths the area is a better guide. For this reason spectrometers are equipped with an integrating device. The numbers of protons determined by integration are indicated by the numbers on the spectra.

Consider the spectrum (Fig. 9.2) of α-chloro propionic acid. This contains three groups of resonances, one at low field, one at 4.45 ppm, and one at 1.75 ppm. The high field doublet is split by spin coupling since the same splitting is observed in the quartet. Thus we have three sorts of proton. Inspection of Fig. 9.1 suggests that these belong to the fragments HC–C, HC(C=O)R, and a hydrogen-bonded proton. The doublet–quartet AX_3 part of the spectrum has a typical vicinal coupling constant of 7 Hz so that we have the fragment $CH_3–CH(CO)R$.

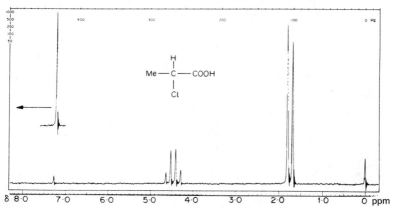

Figure 9.2   60 MHz proton spectrum of α-chloropropionic acid.
(Reproduced by permission of Varian International AG.)

The intensities suggest proton ratios of 3:1:1. If we were given that the
empirical formula is $C_3H_5O_2$ Cl then we could write the structural
formula as $CH_3-CH(CO)OH$ and place the chlorine atom appropriately
to satisfy the valence rules.

   Now apply the same approach to Figs 9.3 to 9.10. The formulae are
grouped in Fig. 9.11 with one extra inserted to reduce the possibility of
analysis by elimination. Bear in mind: (i) that the fluorine resonances
of the fluorine-containing compounds are not visible, though splitting
due to fluorine may be; (ii) that broadened NH proton resonances may
nevertheless cause splitting in vicinal protons; (iii) that the outer lines of
a multiplet with many lines may not be visible (use Pascal's triangle to
check the multiplicity of the apparent quintet of Fig. 9.9); and (iv) that
alcoholic protons usually exchange and are variable in position.

9.2   Determination of the structures of organic molecules using proton and carbon spectra together

We have shown in the previous chapters that the carbon spectra are
capable of yielding much information through a series of quite time
consuming experiments. These facilities are normally reserved for the
more difficult samples and often it will be sufficient to have simply the
broad band proton decoupled spectrum. This gives the chemical shift
information, details of coupling to nuclei other than hydrogen, and a
carbon count, provided all the likely errors in line intensity are taken

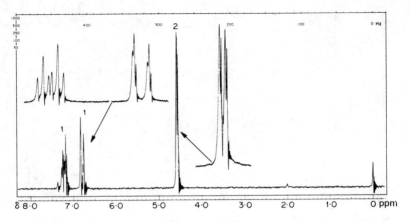

Figure 9.3

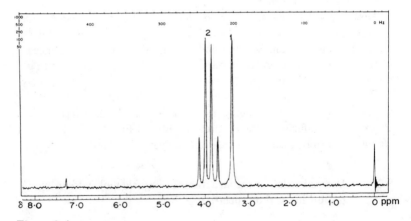

Figure 9.4

Figures 9.3–9.10   60 MHz proton spectra of eight of the substances depicted in Fig. 9.11. Where resonances appear below 8 ppm they have been recorded with the spectrometer scale offset, to bring the resonance onto the paper. (Reproduced by permission of Varian International AG.)

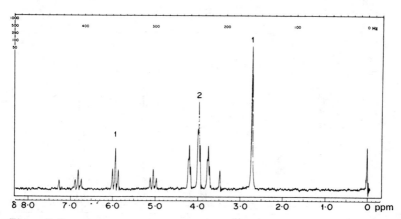

Figure 9.5

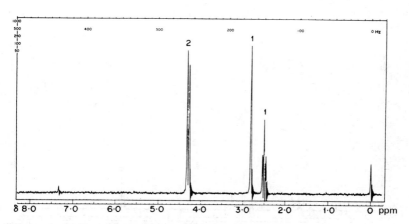

Figure 9.6 (for caption see p.190)

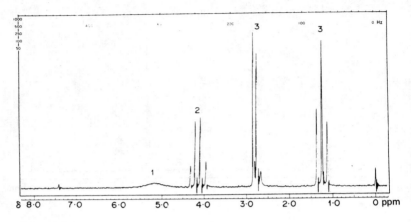

Figure 9.7

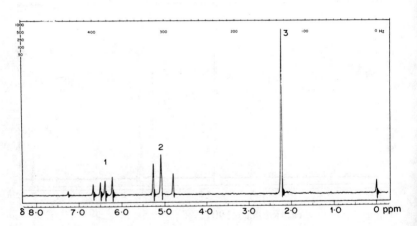

Figure 9.8   (for caption see p. 190)

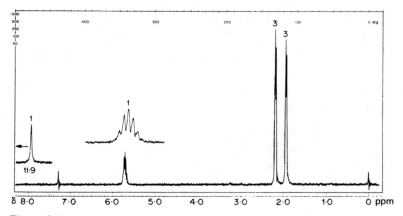

Figure 9.9

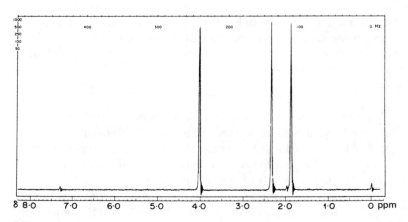

Figure 9.10   (for caption see p. 190)

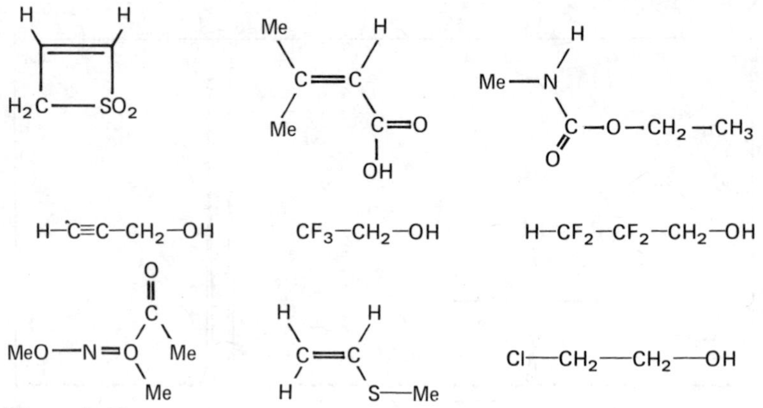

Figure 9.11

into account. It is also certain that the proton spectrum will be available since this is so easy to obtain, and interpretation will be based on the two sets of data taken together. The carbon spectra of course give information about carbon atoms not bonded to hydrogen which is not available in the proton spectra.

The carbon chemical shifts are much more widely dispersed than are the proton shifts. The ranges within which different types of carbon atom resonate are shown in Fig. 9.12. The chemical shift of a given carbon atom in a family of compounds is sensitive to the influence of all four substituents and for alkanes for instance can be predicted using the Grant and Paul rules

$$\delta_i = -2.6 + 9.1n_\alpha + 9.4n_\beta - 2.5n_\gamma + 0.3n_\delta$$

The chemical shift of carbon i can be calculated from the number of directly bonded carbons (n_α) and the number of carbon atoms two (n_β), three (n_γ) and four (n_δ) bonds removed. The chemical shift of methane is -2.6 ppm. Similar rules exist for ethylenic hydrocarbons and substituent effects have been documented.

The use of the two sets of information together is illustrated in Fig. 9.13 for the simple case of ethyl benzene. The 60 MHz proton spectrum contains the unmistakable quartet—triplet pattern due to an ethyl group and five protons resonate in the aromatic region. This is indeed sufficient to give the structure in this case, especially if the formula weight were known. However, we note for the purposes of illustration that there is no structure in the aromatic resonance and we would find that no useful improvement could be obtained even at the highest fields. We therefore turn our attention to the carbon spectrum, also in Fig. 9.13. We find the two carbons of the ethyl group and four aromatic resonances. The one to low field is rather small as would be expected for quaternary carbon. Of the remaining three, two are significantly larger and might arise from two carbons. The pattern has the form to be expected for a mono substituted six membered ring and allows us to over determine the structure of this molecule. All its

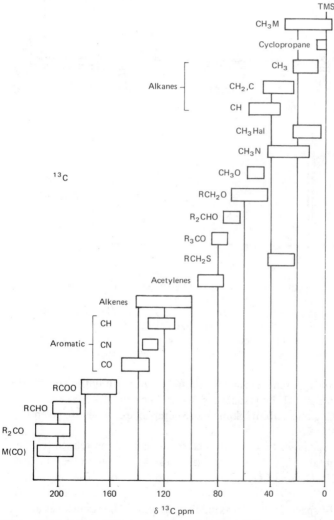

Figure 9.12   Chart of approximate chemical shift ranges of carbon atom nuclei in organic and organometallic compounds. M represents a metal and Hal a halogen.

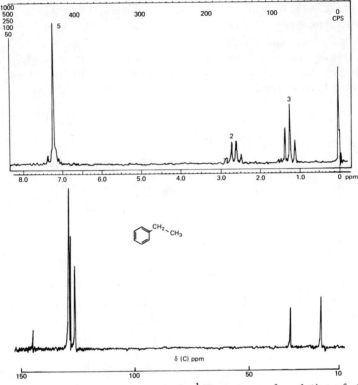

Figure 9.13   The upper trace is the ^{1}H spectrum of a solution of ethyl benzene in CDCl$_3$ obtained 60 MHz and with TMS added as reference. The lower trace is the ^{13}C spectrum obtained at 22.6 MHz with proton broad band decoupling at 90 MHz. No TMS was present in this case, the calibration being based on the deuterium lock frequency. (Upper plot reproduced by permission of Varian International AG.)

features are apparent, though we should note carefully the ambiguities of the intensity of the resonances. Which line should we take as representing one carbon? Some more complex examples are given in Figs 9.14 to 9.17.

Fig. 9.15 shows two carbon spectra of a compound related to that used to obtain Fig. 9.14 but synthesized so as to contain the substituents CH$_3$–, CH$_3$O– and CH$_3$OCO– on the aromatic core. The empirical formula is C$_{16}$H$_{14}$O$_3$N$_2$ and this and the parent compound have very similar UV spectra with a maximum at 360 nm. The resonances are displayed in two groups, 0 to 70 ppm and 95 to 170 ppm. In each group the lower spectrum is with broad band proton irradiation and the upper, noisy one is without and so displays all the carbon–hydrogen couplings, whose values are included on the spectra. The large values

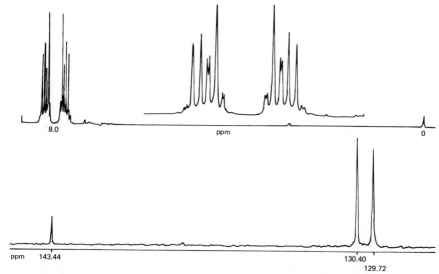

Figure 9.14   The 80 MHz proton spectrum (upper) and 20.1 MHz ^{13}C
spectrum (lower) of the aromatic compound $C_{12}N_2H_8$. The proton
spectrum is diagnostic of an AA′BB′ four spin system in which there
are two pairs of protons with the same chemical shift δ_A, δ_B, but
different coupling constants $J(AB)$, $J(AA′)$, $J(AB′)$, and $J(BB′)$. Only
the three lines are observed in the carbon spectrum. This information
is sufficient to identify the compound, two suggestions appearing below.
(Example provided by A. Römer.)

represent the one bond C–H couplings. Typical values of the longer
range C–H couplings are HCC (^2J) ~ 1, HCCC (^3J) ~ 9 and HCCCC
(^4J) ~ 1 Hz in these aromatic systems. Fig. 9.16 shows the proton
spectrum of the same molecule. The broad lines near 1 ppm are
impurities, the quintet near 2 ppm is the remnant hydrogen in the
deutero-acetone solvent and the singlet at 2.7 ppm is water. The
multiplet at 2.8 ppm is a doublet of doublets and that at 4 ppm is an
unequal doublet. The lower field half of the multiplet near 7.3 ppm
(due to two protons) contains one coupling equal to the larger one
observed in the multiplet at 2.8 ppm, and the broadening in the high
field half can be assigned to the other coupling, though this is
unresolved in the aromatic resonance. The data in the three spectra are
sufficient to allow a full structural assignment to be made, taking into
account the pattern in the proton aromatic region and the long range
C–H couplings.

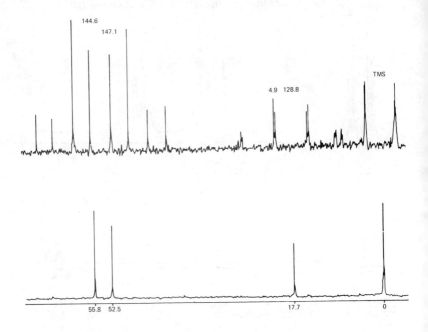

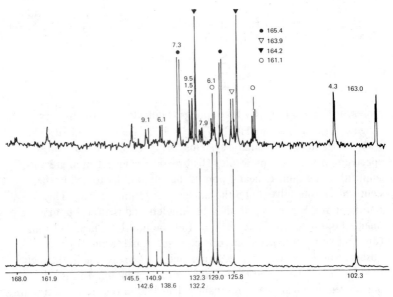

Figure 9.15

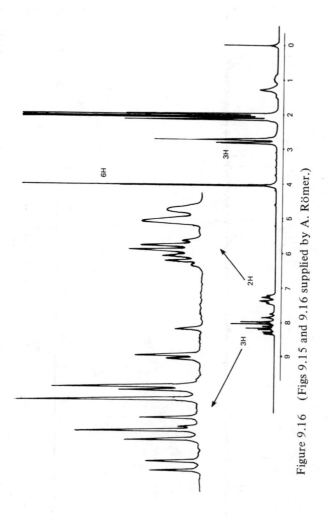

Figure 9.16 (Figs 9.15 and 9.16 supplied by A. Römer.)

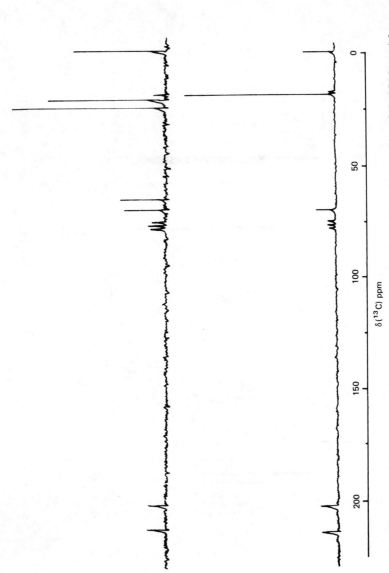

Figure 9.17   The ^{13}C spectra of starting material (lower) and product (upper) in the reaction of C_4SOMe_4 with permaleic acid to give $C_8H_{12}SO_2$. The triplet near 75 ppm is due to the $CDCl_3$ solvent and the singlet at 0 ppm is the TMS reference.

$\delta(^{13}C)$ ppm

The final ^{13}C example shows how the technique was used to determine the result of a synthesis. It was desired to introduce an oxygen atom into the four membered ring of the compound shown to form a lactone and this was attempted by a Baeyer–Villiger oxidation using permaleic acid. The red starting material gave a white product with the correct formula, $C_8H_{12}SO_2$. The proton spectra were trivial, the starting material giving a singlet at 1.35 ppm, a singlet since the four methyl groups are normal to the plane of the ring, and the product, two lines of equal area at 1.51 and 1.65 ppm. Thus the reaction had led to a product in which the two sets of methyl groups had been differentiated. All seemed well until the ^{13}C spectra were obtained.

These are shown in Fig. 9.17. The starting material has resonances due to CH_3-, the methyl substituted ring carbons and the C:S and C:O carbon atoms, as expected. The introduction of an oxygen atom next to the ring carbons would be expected to move their resonances about 25 ppm downfield. In the event, only very small changes are observed, indicating that while the symmetry of the ring has changed, the chemical environment of its atoms has changed very little. Thus the oxygen is attached to the sulphur and has not been inserted into the ring.

9.3   Determination of the conformations of molecules

Cyclohexane is known to exist in the chair configuration, of which there are two forms, a given proton being equatorial in one and axial in the other (Fig. 9.18). Interconversion of the two forms is rapid at room temperature and so the protons experience an average environment and the proton resonance is a sharp singlet. If the rate of interconversion is reduced by cooling, or by fixing the conformation by substitution, or

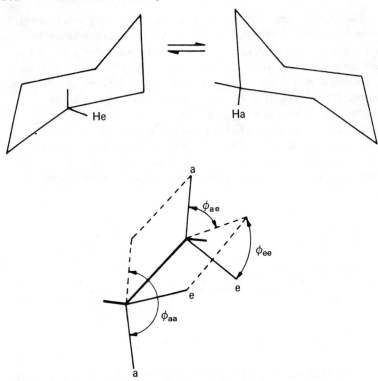

Figure 9.18   Upper: Interconverting chair forms of cyclohexane, C_6H_{12} indicating how one proton changes from an axial (a) to an equatorial (e) position. Lower: A view of carbon—carbon bond of cyclohexane showing the various dihedral angles between the carbon—hydrogen bonds. The hydrogen positions are designated a or e.

by incorporation in a large molecule, the situation becomes much more complex and the individual protons take individual chemical shifts and can show mutual spin—spin coupling. In the $-CH_2-CH_2-$ fragment in Fig. 9.18 we can see that a given proton can be coupled to up to five others and that the magnitude of the coupling will depend upon the dihedral angles ϕ_{aa}, ϕ_{ae} as given by the Karplus relationships (Fig. 3.1).

In the case of the six-membered cyclic molecules of the glycosides the rate of ring flexing is often reduced by the presence of a bulky substituent, which tends to take an equatorial position because of the steric crowding which occurs in the axial position. If the hydroxyl groups are acetylated the OH resonances are eliminated, and clear spectra of the protons on the ring skeleton are obtained. Their chemical

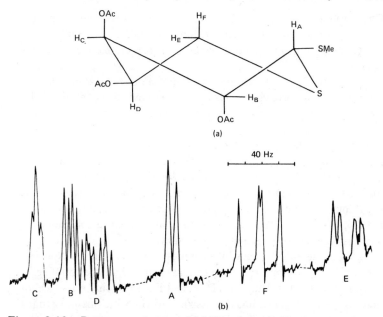

Figure 9.19   Proton spectrum at 90 MHz of the dithioglycoside
$\overline{S\ CH(SMe)CH(OAc)CH(OAc)CH(OAc)CH_2}$. (a) The spectrum (b) is
exhibited as a series of expanded sections to show up the fine structure.
The full spectrum extends over 3.7 ppm. The three high-field lines due
to the four methyl groups in the molecule are omitted.

shifts extend over a large range and the resulting spin coupling patterns
between them are first order and can be used to determine the
conformation of the molecule. This is possible because the dihedral
angle between pairs of vicinal protons is large (near 180°) in the case of
two axial protons but much smaller and near to 60° in the case of two
equatorial or an equatorial and an axial proton (Fig. 9.18). Reference
to the Karplus curves (Fig. 3.1) will show that we would expect the
spin–spin coupling between two axial protons to be much larger than
that between two equatorial protons or between an equatorial and an
axial proton.

Using this rule we can obtain the configuration of the dithioglycoside
whose formula and spectrum are shown in Fig. 9.19. The spectrum can
be assigned to individual protons as follows. The proton H_A is the only
one coupled to a single proton and therefore will be the only one
exhibiting simple doublet splitting. Thus multiplet A arises from H_A.

The coupling constant of 5 Hz is small and must arise from an axial–equatorial or equatorial–equatorial interaction. Since the bulky S Me group will take up an equatorial position then H_A is axial and H_B is equatorial.

H_B is coupled to two protons and therefore its resonance will be a quartet with one spacing of 5 Hz due to coupling to H_A. Multiplet B is the only one which satisfies this condition and measurement of the second splitting indicates that H_B is coupled to H_C by 2.8 Hz.

Looking further around the ring we see that H_D is also a unique proton in that it is the only one coupled to three other protons. Its resonance should therefore consist of a doublet, of doublets, of doublets i.e. eight lines, all of equal height. Multiplet D is the only one satisfying this condition. Measurement gives three coupling constants of 11.4, 4.0, and 2.8 Hz, the first being a large, axial–axial coupling which is repeated only in multiplet F. Multiplet F is a quartet with a second splitting of 13.1 Hz which is repeated in multiplet E. Now two of our protons, H_E and H_F, are a geminal pair and a large coupling constant is expected. Multiplets D, E, and F are the only ones exhibiting large coupling constants but D is assigned to H_D which has no geminal proton. Therefore multiplets E and F arise from the geminal pair. H_D and the proton giving rise to resonance F must both be axial to account for the large vicinal coupling. Resonance F thus must arise from H_F and by elimination resonance E is due to H_E. Measurement of multiplet E indicates that H_E is coupled to H_D by 4.0 Hz, a small value as expected. This leaves one coupling of 2.8 Hz to H_D unaccounted for and this must arise from coupling to H_C. It is a small value and H_C must be equatorial. H_C is coupled to H_B also by 2.8 Hz so that the two centre lines of its quartet overlap and it is observed as a triplet; multiplet C. The coupling constant between H_B and H_C is small, consistent with both being equatorial.

A similar spectral example has already been given in Fig. 8.2 where it will be observed that the equatorial–equatorial, 1–2 coupling is smaller than the other axial–axial couplings.

9.4   Proton homonuclear double resonance studies

9.4.1   As an aid in understanding a spectral feature

Fig. 9.20 shows the structure and spectra of a palladium complex with *trans* carbon–metal bonds. The multiplets are sufficiently separated to make a complete assignment based upon the coupling patterns (AB_2

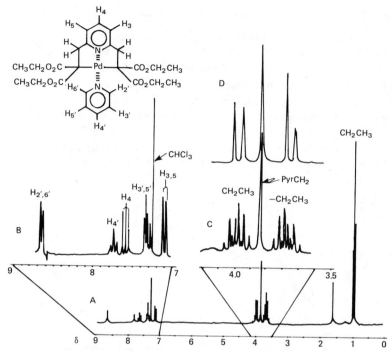

Figure 9.20   200–MHz ^{1}H NMR spectrum (A) of a complex in CDCl$_3$ at 40 °C, expanded aromatic and methylene regions (B, C) and the decoupled methylene region (D). (Reproduced with permission from Newkome *et al.* (1981) *J. Amer. Chem. Soc.*, **103**, 3423.)

and AB$_2$X$_2$ for the pyridine rings) the integral (not shown) and the chemical shifts. There is however a rather strange feature in the region near 4.0 ppm where the CH$_2$ of the 2,6-substituted pyridine is a singlet but the methylene protons of the ethyl side groups give a pair of complex multiplets. The singlet indicates that the molecule has a plane of symmetry and this would normally mean that the methylene protons were equivalent and would appear as a quartet. A double resonance experiment was therefore carried out in which the methyl triplet at 1 ppm was irradiated and the quartet splitting eliminated from the methylene multiplet. The result is an AB type of pattern with a large geminal coupling, which can arise only if the two protons on each methylene carbon have different chemical shifts. Thus rotation of the ethyl group does not result in these two protons attaining the same magnetic environment because there is no molecular plane of symmetry through the bonds attaching them to the rings.

9.4.2   As an aid in solving a complex structure

The protoporphyrin N-methylprotoporphyrin IX(dimethyl ester) has four isomers which differ in the ring which has been N-methylated (Fig. 9.21). The four isomers can be separated by chromatography and have quite different proton spectra which, provided we can assign the resonances to individual protons, can be used to distinguish the isomers. The porphyrin ring system supports an appreciable ring current and an interesting feature of the spectrum is that the *meso* protons, in the position analogous to those in benzene, are moved strongly to low field between 10.0 and 10.5 ppm from TMS, while the N-methyl protons

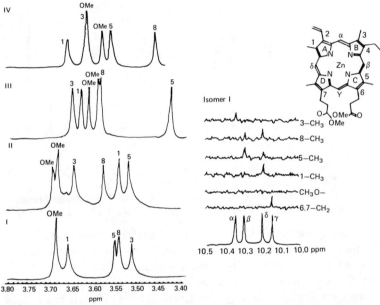

Figure 9.21   Proton spectra of N-methylprotoporphyrin IX(dimethyl ester) zinc complex. The formula is inset top right without the N-methyl group, which may be on any of the four rings A—D. The *meso* protons are labelled with Greek letters. Their normal and Overhauser difference spectra are shown on the right for isomer I and the normal spectra of the ring methyl substituents of all four isomers are shown on the left. The methyl resonances are assigned for each isomer by finding their NOE on the *meso* protons and the position of N-methylation in each isomer deduced by finding which isomer has which methyl signal shifted anomalously high field. The *meso* protons were assigned initially by a partial deuteration experiment. (Reproduced with permission from Kuntze and Ortiz de Montellane (1981) *J. Amer. Chem. Soc.,* **103**, 4225.)

inside the current loop are found high field of TMS at −4.6 ppm.

The first stage in the investigation of the spectra was to make use of the knowledge that the rate of deuterium exchange at the *meso* sites of such molecules decreased in the order $\gamma > \delta > \beta > \alpha$. The sites were thus partially deuterated and the spectra obtained. The line intensities decreased in the order that the rate of exchange increased and so allowed the four *meso* resonances to be assigned for each isomer. These assignments were partially confirmed by a relaxation measurement of the *meso* protons. The results for isomer I were:

site	α	β	γ	δ
T_1/s	1.16	1.10	0.65	1.04

The γ site has the shortest relaxation time because it is influenced by two propionic acid side chains.

The next step is to make use of the fact that the N-methylation of the ring in such compounds causes the chemical shift of the C-methyl substituents to be displaced up-field. If we can identify which methyl resonance belongs to which methyl substituent and find the one at anomalously high field, then we have the answer to our problem. Since the molecule is a rigid one, it is ideal for an Overhauser experiment as the proton–proton distances are well defined. Each of the methyl resonances was irradiated in turn while a spectrum was obtained and a normal spectrum (no irradiation) was then subtracted. The difference spectrum then contains only the NOE enhancements, which become particularly noticeable (Fig. 9.21). For isomer I we see that γ is affected only by irradiation of the propionic acid side chain methylene protons, δ is affected strongly by two which must be the 1- and 8-Me, the proximity of the shift of the last to that of a further Me indicating that it is the 8 substituent. The irradiation of the other of this pair affects β and confirms that it is the 5-Me. Finally, irradiating the highest field Me affects α and the assignment of all the methyl groups is completed. Identification of the 3-methyl groups in all four isomers by the same procedure confirms that in I the 3-Me is at the highest field so that I is N-methylated in the ring marked B.

9.4.3   As an aid in determining the shape of a flexible side chain

The cobalt complex shown on Fig. 9.22 has four equatorial methyl groups, all with the same chemical shift, and a propyl group in close proximity to them. The 400 MHz proton spectrum of the propyl part of the spectrum is shown in the figure (lower spectrum) and the NOE

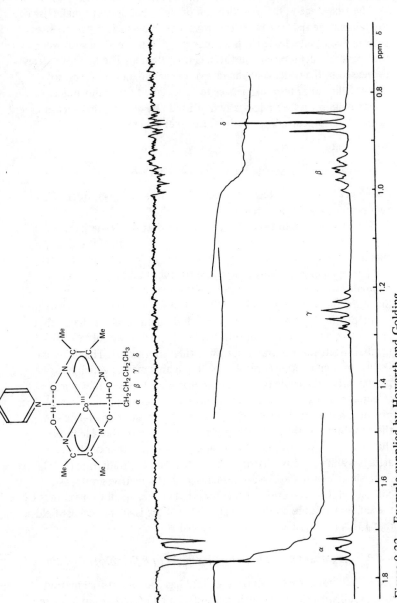

Figure 9.22   Example supplied by Howarth and Golding.

difference spectrum obtained while irradiating the equatorial methyl groups. It is clear from the integral traces of the latter that two of the multiplets show an NOE and two do not. The obvious disturbance at the position of the triplet, which must be due to a small frequency shift, integrates to zero. If we can assign the individual propyl resonances then we will know which are nearest to the equatorial methyls. The triplet to high field is obviously due to the CH_3-. The sextet at 1.25 ppm is the γ CH_2, coupled to five protons and the quintet must arise from the next methylene group along the chain. The α methylene also gives a triplet, though distorted due to second order effects which probably indicate that there is some restriction of rotation at this end of the molecule. We then see that only the groups near the cobalt suffer an NOE and that the propyl chain must be normal to the dimethylglyoxime plane and not bent over as depicted on the formula.

9.5   The determination of the structures of transition metal complexes

A vast array of transition metal complexes is now known in which the central metal atom is bonded to several of a possible multitude of monodentate ligands, e.g. carbonyl, CO; hydride, H; a phosphine, $PRR'R''$; a halide; or an organic group. Complexes are also formed with bidentate ligands such as ethylenediamine and with unsaturated organic systems *via* the π-bonds. The stereochemistry of such complexes offers considerable possibility of variation and NMR has been found to be invaluable in deciding just how the ligands are arranged around the metal atom. The NMR spectrum of a ligand is usually that expected to arise from its structure though the chemical shifts of the resonances of the free and complexed ligand and the coupling constants will be different. There are however a number of other features which are of use to the chemist, for instance the very high field shift of metal hydride protons is diagnostic of their presence and spin coupling may be observed between ligands or between ligand and metal if the metal has a magnetically active isotope (Fig. 9.23).

Cis—trans effects in complexes are manifested also in their NMR spectra. Ligands are affected much more strongly by groupings *trans* to them and are relatively indifferent to *cis* groupings. Thus metal—ligand coupling constants are dependent upon the nature of the group or atom *trans* to the ligand. For instance, in complexes of the type depicted in

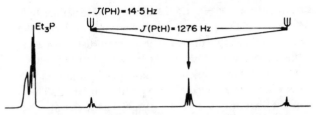

Figure 9.23   60 MHz proton spectrum of *trans* Pt HCl(PEt$_3$)$_2$ in benzene. The ethyl resonance of the phosphine ligands appear at low field while the hydride resonance is 16.9 ppm high field of TMS. The hydride resonance is split into a triplet by coupling to the two equivalent phosphorus atoms, $^2J(P–H) = 14.5$ Hz and has identical platinum satellites due to coupling to the 33.7% of ^{195}Pt present. (After Chatt and Shaw (1962) *J. Chem. Soc.*, 5075, with permission.)

Fig. 9.23, $^1J(^{195}\text{Pt}–^{31}\text{P})$ is ca. 1400 Hz in the position *trans* to H and ca. 3500 Hz *trans* to Cl. Chemical shifts are determined principally by *trans* ligands and spin–spin coupling is strong between trans pairs of ligands, weak between *cis* pairs. This difference means that study of the methyl proton resonances of tertiary methyl phosphines in complexes containing several such ligands provides a very useful guide to their stereochemistry. Pairs of methyl phosphines can be considered as forming the four spin system

$$\text{H} \ldots \text{P} \ldots (\text{Metal}) \ldots \text{P}' \ldots \text{H}'$$

in which for simplicity only one proton is considered per phosphine and the carbon atoms are omitted. All nuclei have $I = \frac{1}{2}$. The primed and unprimed atoms are not magnetically equivalent since $J(P–H)$ and $J(P–H')$ are not the same. Since both P and P' and H and H' have the same chemical shifts a second-order spectrum results. This can be simply analysed by dividing the full spectrum into subspectra as follows:

(i) When both phosphorus spins are +. The two hydrogen atoms are isochronous and give rise to a singlet.

(ii) Similarly when both phosphorus spins are − another singlet is obtained. The separation between the two singlets is $|J(H–P) + J(H–P')|$, its magnitude depending upon the relative signs of the two couplings. Thus the spectrum always contains a 1:1 doublet.

(iii) When the two phosphorus atoms have different (opposite) spins the two protons are no longer isochronous and can exhibit spin coupling. However $J(H–H')$ is usually negligibly small but virtual coupling occurs via the strong H–P and P–P' interactions such that an

AB spectrum results with each half based on one of the singlets and with an apparent coupling equal to $J(P–P')$ (Fig. 9.24a). If $J(P–P')$ is small, i.e. $J(P–P') \ll |J(H–P) + J(H–P')|$ then the lines of the AB sub-spectrum are close to the singlets and may not be resolved, so that a deceptively simple doublet results (Fig. 9.24b). Alternatively if $J(P–P')$ is large so that $J(P–P') > |J(H–P) + J(H–P')|$ then a closely coupled AB sub-spectrum is obtained with the two central lines close

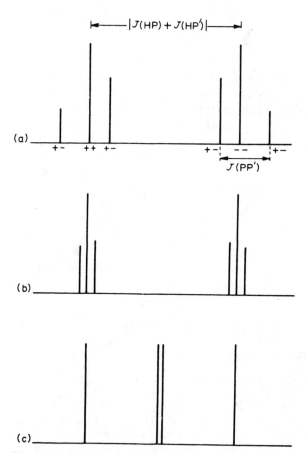

Figure 9.24   Proton spectra due to the two protons in the four spin system H . . . P . . . Metal . . . P$'$ . . . H$'$. In (b) $J(P–P') \ll |J(P–H) + J(P–H')|$ and the spectrum is essentially a doublet while in (c) $J(P–P') > |(J(P–H) + J(P–H')|$ and the spectrum approximates a 1:2:1 triplet. The small signs indicate the PP$'$ spin combinations giving rise to the different sub-spectra.

together and containing virtually all the sub-spectral intensity (Fig. (Fig. 9.24c). In this case a deceptively simple 1:2:1 triplet results which appears to indicate that the protons are equally coupled to each phosphorus. Thus *trans* pairs of methyl phosphines give rise to a methyl triplet whereas *cis* pairs of phosphines give a methyl doublet. An example of a *trans* complex is given in Fig. 9.25 (the different *cis* and *trans* couplings are exemplified in Fig. 9.45). The P—methyl and Pt—methyl resonance multiplicities give the same information in this case. The latter also demonstrate how the arrangement of ligands can be deduced from the patterns seen in the NMR spectra.

Metal complexes can also be formed with a variety of unsaturated compounds. The π-electrons of the unsaturated bonds form bonds to the metal and in so doing their bond order is reduced. Olefinic protons for instance are normally descreened but when a π-complex is formed the bond anisotropy changes and we see a high field shift. Thus if 1, 4-dimethyl naphthaline is complexed with chromium tricarbonyl (Fig. 9.26) the chromium can bond into the π-system of either ring and two products are obtained. The spectrum of each consists of a methyl singlet (not shown) a singlet for the isolated, isochronous C protons at positions 2 and 3, and an $[AB]_2$ spectrum for the 5, 6, 7, and 8 protons. These last two features can be clearly observed for both compounds in Fig. 9.26 where it will be seen that for the predominant complex the C singlet is low field of the $[AB]_2$ multiplet so that complexing has occurred *via* the unsubstituted ring, whereas in the minor component the C singlet is high field of the $[AB]_2$ multiplet, indicating complexing in the methyl substituted ring.

Figure 9.25   The 100 MHz proton spectrum of the high field, methyl region of the complex $PtBrMe(PMe_2R)_2$, where the group R is 2,4-dimethoxyphenyl attached to phosphorus at the 1 position. The lower spectrum is obtained normally and the upper one with irradiation of [31]P. Both the P bonded and Pt bonded methyl groups show the characteristic 1:4:1 triplet due to coupling to the 33.7% abundant [195]Pt. The Pt bonded methyl resonates close to TMS and is split into a 1:2:1 triplet by the two phosphorus atoms. This is in fact sufficient in this case to identify the complex as a *trans* complex since *cis* phosphines would couple differently to this methyl group and give a doublet of doublets. We note however, that the P methyl groups also give a 1:2:1 triplet even though they cannot be coupled equally to the two phosphorus atoms and can recognize virtual coupling of the type described in the previous figure. [31]P irradiation as expected, removes all these features and leaves only the Pt—H coupling. (Example supplied by Professor B. L. Shaw.)

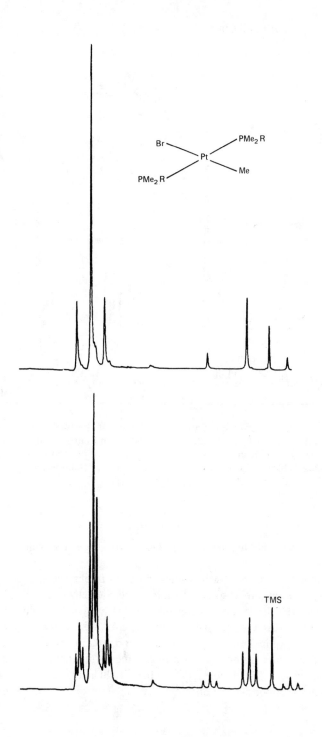

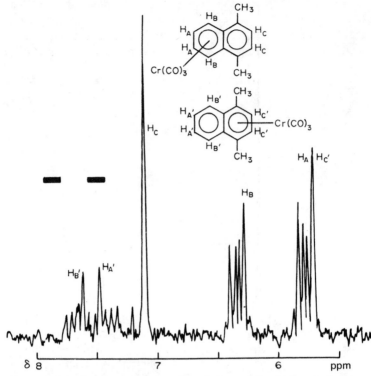

Figure 9.26   Proton spectrum of a mixture of the two complexes formed between 1, 4-dimethyl naphthalene and chromium tricarbonyl. The two sets of resonances are differentiated by primed letters. The two black bars indicate the region in which naphthalene resonates. (After Deubzer *et al.* (1969) *J. Organometall. Chem.*, 7, 289, with permission.)

9.6   Variable temperature studies of some dynamic systems

Variable temperature NMR studies enable us to observe and measure the changes in rate of some dynamic process which affects the NMR spectra. The first example here concerns the behaviour of aluminium trimethyl. This was believed to be dimeric Al_2Me_6 with two bridging and four terminal methyl groups but at room temperature its proton NMR spectrum is simply a sharp singlet suggesting that all six methyls are equivalent. This is contrary to what would be expected since the bridging methyls are in a different environment to the terminal methyl groups. In cyclohexane solution however it was found that as the temperature was reduced the methyl resonance broadened and separated into two singlets of intensity ratio 1:2, arising respectively from the bridging and terminal methyl groups. The two sorts of methyl group are thus interchanging roles rapidly on the NMR time scale at room temperature. The activation energy for exchange was calculated from the exchange rates obtained from the line-shapes and was found to be 65 kJ mol^{-1}. This is probably similar to the energy of dissociation of the dimer in solution so that exchange may proceed via dissociation of the dimer. It was also possible to conclude from these spectra that the carbon atom of the bridging methyl groups probably forms the bridge link and that none of its hydrogens were directly involved, since these were all equivalent down to the lowest temperatures (Fig. 9.27).

A second field of study where NMR has been of assistance is that of σ-cyclopentadienyl metal complexes (Fig. 9.28). The room temperature proton spectrum of these compounds is a singlet and so does not in itself differentiate them from the π-cyclopentadienyl complexes where the metal is placed above a face of the ring and is equally bound to all five carbons, as in ferrocene. As the temperature is reduced however the spectrum of a σ bonded ring broadens and splits into three separate peaks corresponding to the three types of proton in the σ compound (Fig. 9.28). This behaviour is of course indicative of rapid exchange at room temperature with the metal attached successively to each ring carbon atom thus averaging the proton environments to a single one. The exchange can take place in one of three ways: (i) by 1:2 hops, i.e. the metal moves always from one carbon atom to either of the adjacent two; (ii) by 1:3 hops where the metal always moves to either of the next but one carbons; or (iii) randomly with processes (i) and (ii) of equal probability. The spectra in Fig. 9.28b allow us to choose which process is occurring. Why this is so is best seen by reference to Fig. 9.28c. This indicates that when a 1:2 hop occurs an A spin becomes A, the other A spin becomes B, a B spin becomes A and so on. Now the A and B spins resonate close together so that when an A ↔ B interchange occurs there is only a small degree of frequency uncertainty introduced. The X resonance however is well removed from both A and B so that when an A ↔ X or B ↔ X interchange occurs the frequency uncertainty, and consequent line broadening, is much greater. When an 1:2 hop occurs only B interchanges with X whereas when a 1:3 hop occurs only A interchanges with X. Thus in the case of 1:2 hops we expect the B resonance to be broader than the A resonance while if 1:3 hops occur then the A resonance will be the broader. If

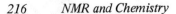

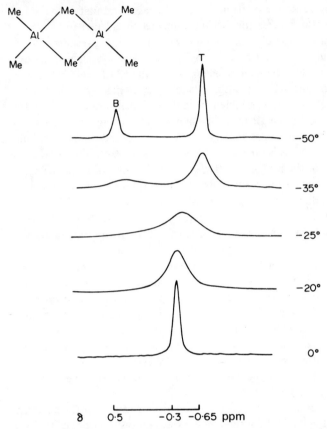

Figure 9.27   Proton spectra at several temperatures of aluminium trimethyl dimer dissolved in cyclohexane. The terminal methyl groups (T) resonate high field of TMS but the involvement of the bridging methyls in further bonding results in their being descreened (b) (After Ramey, O'Brien, Hasegawa and Borchert (1965) *J. Phys. Chem.*, **69**, 3418–23.)

random hops occur the broadening will be equal. Reference to Fig. 9.28b shows that the A and B resonances are non-symmetrical, especially between −41° and −54° and that the random hop mechanism is immediately ruled out. Choice of the 1:2 or 1:3 mechanism depends upon correctly assigning which of the two low field resonances is A or B. Currently there is some controversy over this for the copper compound shown, but for the complex (σ-C_5H_5) RuH(π-C_5H_5), which contains both a σ- and a π-bonded ring and

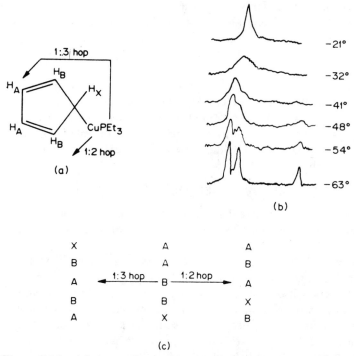

Figure 9.28   (a) A σ-cyclopentadienyl compound. The protons form an [AB]₂ X system and should give rise to three resonances. (b) The proton spectrum at several temperatures of σ-cyclopentadienyl (triethyl phosphine) copper (*I*). The X proton is found to high field and the olefinic A and B protons to low field. Note the asymmetry in the low field region between −41° and −54°. (c) When a metal hop occurs the hydrogens interchange positions in different ways depending upon whether a 1:2 or a 1:3 hop is made (after Whitsides and Fleming, (1967) *J. Amer. Chem. Soc.* **89**, 2855 with permission.)

whose σ-ring spectrum shows similar temperature dependence to the copper compound, it has been established from the structure observed in the resonances at the lowest temperature which of the olefinic resonances couples most strongly to H_X and therefore which is H_B. The results indicate the 1:2 hops as the correct mechanism of exchange in this case.

The hydration complexes formed by ions undergo rapid exchange processes, in this case between molecules of the bulk solvent and of the hydration complex. The rates of exchange for the alkali metal salt solutions are too fast for NMR to be able to see separate resonances for bulk solvent and for solvation solvent, but for the smaller, more highly charged ions such as Be^{2+} and Al^{3+} the rates of exchange are much slower and the technique has made considerable contributions to our knowledge.

The greatest amount of data has been obtained for the aluminium (III) ion. The hydration complex $Al(H_2O)_n^{3+}$ contains three magnetically active nuclei, ^1H, ^{17}O, and ^{27}Al, and all three have been used in a variety of studies concerned with determination of the value of n and of the rates of exchange of hydration water. Because of the hydrolysis reaction of the ion:

$$H_2O + Al(H_2O)_n^{3+} \rightleftharpoons Al(H_2O)_{n-1}(OH)^{2+} + H_3O^+$$

there was reason to believe that the water oxygen and hydrogens exchange at different rates so that ^1H and ^{17}O NMR might give different results.

When the ^{17}O resonance is observed (using ^{17}O enriched material) only a single line can be seen due to bulk and solvation water. If a paramagnetic salt is added with a cation having a short-lived hydration complex then the bulk water all rapidly comes under the influence of the ion and its unpaired electrons and suffers an average contact shift, whereas water bound to Al^{3+} does not. Separate bulk and hydration water resonances can then be observed (Fig. 9.29).

Comparison of the areas under the two peaks, together with a knowledge of the water and aluminium content of the solution, allows the value of n to be calculated. This is invariably found to be near 6.0. Raising the temperature causes changes in line-shape which can be used to calculate rates of exchange. This gives the rate constant for oxygen exchange as $k_O = 0.13 \text{ s}^{-1}$ at $25°$.

The proton resonance of an aluminium chloride solution is also a singlet at room temperature. Fortunately the salt is very soluble so that its saturated solution has a considerably depressed freezing point. This allows the solution to be cooled to $-47°$ at which temperature separate resonances are seen for bulk and bound water protons. Variable temperature experiments enable the rate constant for proton exchange to be calculated and this is found to be, $k_H \approx 10^5 \text{ s}^{-1}$ at $25°$. Thus the exchange rates of oxygen and hydrogen differ by several orders of magnitude.

The ^{27}Al resonance of these solutions is a narrow singlet. This provides further proof that the ion is symmetrical around the aluminium, as would be the case for octahedral $Al(H_2O)_6^{3+}$. An

$$H_2O^* \text{ (bulk)} + Co^{2+} (H_2O)_x \rightleftharpoons H_2O + Co^{2+}(H_2O)_{x-1} (H_2O^*)$$

^{17}O normal ^{17}O contact
    chemical   shift
    shift

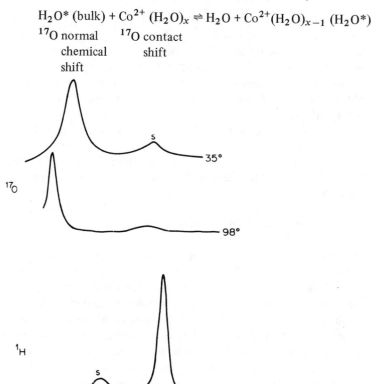

Figure 9.29   Upper: ^{17}O spectra of aqueous $AlCl_3$ with added Co^{2+}. The bulk water is shifted to low field. Raising the temperature increases the rate of oxygen exchange and broadens the resonance of the bound water. (After Connick and Fiat (1963) *J. Chem. Phys.*, **39**, 1349, with permission.)
Lower: ^1H spectrum of concentrated (3M) aqueous $AlCl_3$ at $-47°$. The water in the solvation complex is seen 4.2 ppm to low field of the bulk water. (After Schuster and Fratiello (1967) *J. Chem. Phys.*, **47**, 1554, with permission.) Comparison of the areas of the two peaks in each spectrum allows the hydration number to be calculated and is always near 6.0. s represents the resonance due to solvation water in each case.

unsymmetrical complex with *n* equal to 5 or 7 would have a line broadened by quadrupolar relaxation.

It has been shown similarly that the beryllium cation is tetra-coordinate and exists as tetrahedral $Be(H_2O)_4^{2+}$. In addition it was found that the hydrolysis products could be detected in the proton spectra and that it was possible to follow hydrolysis, both the auto hydrolysis that occurs in the pure salt solution and that caused by added base (Fig. 9.30). Integration of the resonances allowed the number of water molecules coordinated to Be in each species to be obtained and this showed that the cations $Be(H_2O)_4^{2+}$, $(H_2O)_3Be(OH)$-$Be(H_2O)_3^{3+}$ and $[Be(H_2O)_2(OH)]_3^{3+}$ were present as had previously been inferred indirectly from pH titration studies. The ^9Be resonance in all solutions was sharp and showed no chemical shift, consistent with the beryllium being always regularly tetrahedrally coordinated by four oxygen ligands. Another example of an exchanging system will be found on p. 246.

9.7   Lanthanide-induced shifts – shift reagents

We have just seen how the contact shift phenomenon can be used to cause favourable chemical shifts in the study of aqueous salt solutions. Essentially we are using the large magnetic moment of the unpaired electron to produce the shift and are relying on rapid exchange to minimize the relaxation field of the electron at the water oxygens, which stay well removed from the ion for the major part of the time. Thus we avoid too much line broadening of the water resonance.

The effects of paramagnetic species are commonly used to simplify the spectra of organic compounds. A lanthanide shift reagent is an octahedral complex of a lanthanide element (Eu, Dy, Pr or Yb) with a ligand chosen among other things to make the complex soluble in organic solvents, and this is dissolved in a solution of the compound. The lanthanides are capable of assuming higher coordination numbers than six so that if the organic molecule possesses a suitable coordination site (e.g. O or N) it can interact with the complex. This produces an average pseudo contact shift of the protons in the organic molecule which can be very large. For instance the normal spectrum of pentanol is found low field of TMS and consists of a triplet due to the methylene protons adjacent to the alcohol group and two groups containing a series of overlapping lines due to the remaining protons which all have similar chemical shifts. If a praseodymium complex is added (Fig. 9.31) resonances all move upfield of TMS and each become separated sufficiently to give first-order spectra. Alternatively if a europium complex is used the contact shift is down field.

A second example concerns a project to produce an optically active form of hexanol deuterated at the α carbon atom. This was to be achieved using an optically active reducing agent. In order to determine

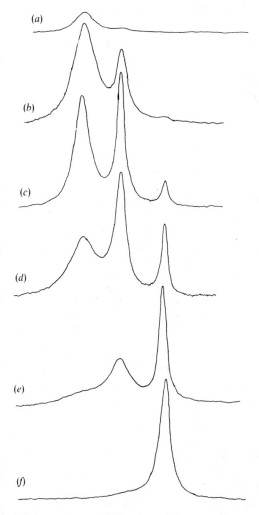

Figure 9.30   220 MHz proton NMR spectra of $BeCl_2$ solutions, pure
(a) and hydrolysed by adding Na_2CO_3 so that the ratio [Na]/[Be] was
(b) 0.12 (c) 0.25 (d) 0.4 (e) 0.65 and (f) 0.92. The spectra were run at
about $-50°$ to slow the water exchange sufficiently to observe
separate resonances for each cation. The lowest field line is due to the
non-hydrolysed cation and is 4 ppm low field of the free water
resonance (not shown). The central line is due to Be_2OH^{3+} and the
high field one to $(BeOH)_3^{3+}$, 1.27 ppm from the lowest field line.
(Reproduced with permission from Akitt and Duncan (1980) *J. Chem.
Soc. Faraday I*, **76**, 2212.)

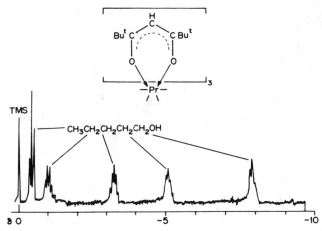

Figure 9.31   The paramagnetic complex tris (2,2,6,6-tetramethyl heptane-3, 5-dionato)-praseodymium has three bulky tridentate ligands surrounding the metal in such a way that it is octahedrally coordinated by oxygen. Only one of the ligands is shown above. Molecules with lone pairs of electrons also approach the paramagnetic metal since the lanthanide can attain coordination numbers greater than six. Their protons can thus interact with the unpaired electrons on the metal and undergo contact shifts. In the case of n-pentanol a first-order spectrum is obtained (Bu^t—represents (CH$_3$)$_3$C— i.e. the *t*-butyl group. This type of ligand is used because it renders the ions soluble in organic solvents). (After Briggs *et al.* (1970) *J. Chem. Soc. Chem. Commun.*, 749, with permission.)

whether optically active products had been formed the 400 MHz proton spectra were obtained in the presence of an optically active lanthanide complex. This produces slightly different chemical shift effects in the different handed products and enables it to be established that racemic forms have been produced and then to follow their preferential production (Fig. 9.32).

Figure 9.32   The 400 MHz proton spectra of the CHD group in various samples of the optically active hexanol, C$_5$H$_{11}$CHDOH, made using an optically active reducing agent. The two optical isomers are detected and distinguished by obtaining the spectra in the presence of an optically active lanthanide complex of europium and a hexafluoro-propyl camphorate (see formula) which induces slightly different shifts in molecules of the same or different sense of activity. The spectra were obtained with selective decoupling of the C$_5$H$_{11}$ protons but remain broad due to coupling to the single deuteron and perhaps some remnant of coupling to the protons and also due to the relaxation effects of the paramagnetic centre. Peak resolution was improved by applying

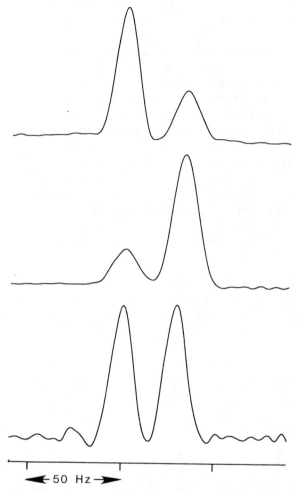

← 50 Hz →

resolution enhancement and this accounts for the rather square
appearance of the peaks. The lower trace shows the racemic mixture,
the centre trace the spectrum obtained when having used the chiral
reducing agent of one hand, and the upper trace that obtained with the
mirror image chiral reducing agent. The complex was:

(Example supplied by B. E. Mann.)

9.8   Significance of carbon-13 relaxation times

Knowledge of the relaxation times of individual carbon atoms in molecules is useful in the first place because it may help in the assignment of carbon resonances. The relaxation time is roughly inversely proportional to the number of hydrogen atoms directly bonded to the carbon atom and allows CH, CH_2 and CH_3 groups to be distinguished. This of course assumes that the relaxation mechanism is dipole–dipole in each case, a condition which can be verified by a nuclear Overhauser measurement. Because relaxation is also determined by the rate of molecular motion, the T_1 values can also tell us a great deal about the way a molecule is moving in solution, and even about differential motion within the same molecule. The individual ^{13}C T_1 values in some molecules are marked on their formulae in Fig. 9.33. The NOEs are generally about 2 except for the

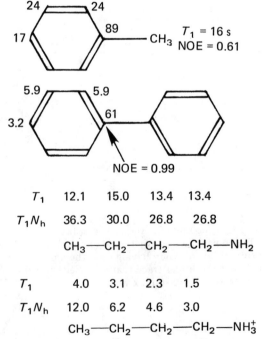

T_1	12.1	15.0	13.4	13.4
$T_1 N_h$	36.3	30.0	26.8	26.8

$$CH_3\text{---}CH_2\text{---}CH_2\text{---}CH_2\text{---}NH_2$$

T_1	4.0	3.1	2.3	1.5
$T_1 N_h$	12.0	6.2	4.6	3.0

$$CH_3\text{---}CH_2\text{---}CH_2\text{---}CH_2\text{---}NH_3^+$$

Figure 9.33   Carbon-13 relaxation times in some molecules. The sample temperatures were all 38°. The aromatic compounds were dissolved in d_6-acetone (ca. 85% solute) and the butyl derivatives were dissolved in D_2O. Fig. 7.2 gives figures for biphenyl in $CDCl_3$.

quaternary carbon in biphenyl and the methyl carbon in toluene. The dipole–dipole mechanism therefore operates predominantly in all but these cases. In the case of toluene, the quaternary carbon has a very long T_1 and the CH carbons relax more efficiently but at different rates. This occurs because the molecular reorientation is anisotropic and the 2 and 3 carbons reorient more often than does the 4 carbon. The rotation of the methyl group is however so fast that the spin–rotation mechanism comes into play and the relaxation time is actually shortened, instead of increased by this motion. Anisotropy in the motion of biphenyl causes similar behaviour in the protonated carbon T_1 values and the quaternary carbon also shows some spin–rotation interaction. Propylamine relaxation times show that segmental motion increases along the alkyl chain, especially if the T_1 values are multiplied by N_h, the number of hydrogen atoms bonded directly to each carbon. The effect increases dramatically if the amino group is protonated to give an end group which is in effect a solvated ion interacting with the solvent.

Part B The use of the other nuclear resonances

Because of the very large number of organic compounds studied by chemists, proton and carbon spectra are those most commonly encountered. They formed the core of Part A and the only others mentioned there were ^{9}Be, ^{17}O, and ^{27}Al. There are many more magnetically active nuclei and we will now survey a small selection of the results which have been obtained with them. Examples involving these nuclei can be expected to increase dramatically in number in the future as the new, multinuclear, high field spectrometers become more widely available. Examples are presented in the order of the groups of the periodic table. Some of the nuclei are relatively little used while others, particularly ^{11}B, ^{19}F and ^{31}P, have proved to be important sources of information and have their own extensive literature.

9.9   Main group I

9.9.1   The lithium-7 resonance

The lithium alkyls have been extensively studied using the ^{7}Li resonance ($I = \frac{3}{2}$). They undergo rapid exchange reactions at room temperature and resolved spectra are best obtained at reduced temperatures. A particularly striking example of this has been the use of ^{7}Li NMR to determine the structure of methyl lithium. This is a tetramer $(LiMe)_4$ but its structure was previously uncertain. The problem was solved by preparing samples containing 25 to 50% ^{13}C-enriched methyl groups. At $-80°$ ^{7}Li septets due to carbon-lithium spin coupling were resolved (Fig. 9.34). The structure of the tetramer is based on a tetrahedron of lithium atoms with the carbon atoms placed symmetrically above each face of the tetrahedron and bridging all three lithium atoms. Each lithium atom can spin couple equally to the three adjacent carbon atoms, ^1J $(^7Li-^{13}C) = 15$ Hz, and the ^{7}Li multiplicity depends upon the number of these which are the ^{13}C isotope. Thus three ^{12}C give a singlet, two ^{12}C and one ^{13}C a doublet, one ^{12}C and two ^{13}C a 1:2:1 triplet and three ^{13}C a 1:4:4:1 quartet. These multiplets interlace to give a septet whose line intensities depend upon the ^{13}C enrichment and with a separation equal to half the coupling constant. This is shown diagrammatically in Fig. 9.34 together with two ^{7}Li spectra of 25 and 50% ^{13}C enriched materials.

9.9.2   The sodium-23 resonance

In general the rates of exchange in solutions containing the alkali metal ions are very fast and only one resonance is observed, even at the lowest temperatures possible for the solvent. The chemical shift depends upon concentration, counter ion and solvent but since the exchange involves many solvate environments the interpretation of such shifts is difficult, there usually being far too many variables to fit meaningfully to a featureless shift—concentration correlation, although qualitative conclusions about the presence of ion pairing can sometimes be made. In the case of the study of the complexes formed by the alkali metals with cryptands it has, however, been found that exchange is sufficiently slow for separate metal signals to be observed (Fig. 9.35) Examples are now known for complexes with lithium and potassium also using ^{7}Li and ^{39}K spectroscopy, respectively. The average lifetime of a sodium atom in a particular environment obtained by line fitting to Fig. 9.35 varies with temperature as follows:

Temperature (°C)	75	65	56	51	44	34
τ (ms)	0.20	0.20	0.39	0.59	0.99	1.67

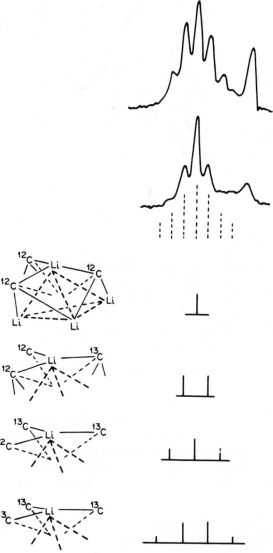

Figure 9.34 The ^{7}Li resonance of ^{13}C-enriched methyl lithium at $-80°$. The high field singlet is a marker due to Li. The upper trace is from a 50% ^{13}C enriched sample and the lower is from a 25% enriched sample. The latter contains more of the molecules with lithium adjacent to three ^{12}C atoms and so has the relatively more intense centre singlet. The stick diagram shows how the septet originates. (After McKeever *et al.* (1969) *J. Amer. Chem. Soc.*, **91**, 1057 with permission.)

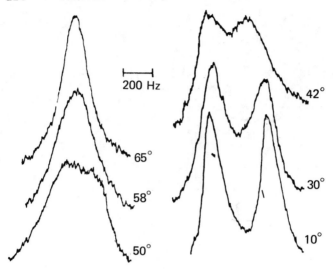

Figure 9.35 ^{23}Na spectra of a solution of NaBr and the cryptand $N(C_2H_4OC_2H_4OC_2H_4)_3N$ in 2:1 mole ratio in ethylenediamine. The solution contains Na^+ solvated by the solvent or complexed by the cryptand and exchange is slow enough for two resonances to be observed separated by 24.3 ppm. The resonances coalesce on heating and the variation of the rate of exchange with temperature is given in the text. (After Ceraso and Dye (1973) *J. Amer. Chem. Soc.*, **95**, 4432 with permission.)

9.10   Main group II

A mention of the use of ^{9}Be has already been made. Otherwise the metals in this group have been relatively little studied due to their poor receptivities. Because of the importance of Ca and Mg in biology considerable efforts are being put into their spectroscopy with the intention of monitoring the way they interact with biological substrates.

9.11   Main group III

9.11.1   The boron-11 resonance

The structure of diborane B_2H_6 was a problem which excited interest for many years and work with this compound led eventually to the concept of the multicentre bond with hydrogen acting as a bridging atom. The NMR spectra of diborane are entirely consistent with the double bridged structure. Fig. 9.36 shows spectra obtained using isotopically nearly pure $^{11}B_2H_6$ which gives a clearer pattern than

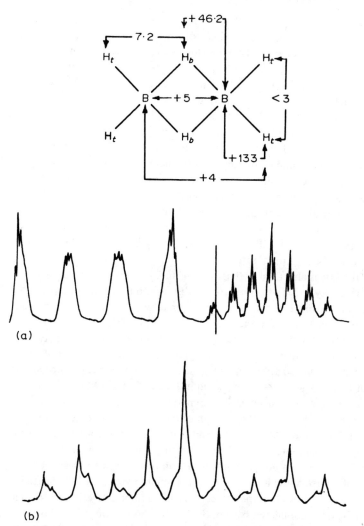

Figure 9.36   The low temperature proton 100 MHz (a), and boron−11 19.25 MHz (b) spectra of diborane, B_2H_6, which was isotopically virtually pure in ^{11}B. The sharp vertical line in (a) is TMS. The terminal proton quartet is low field of this line and the bridge proton septet of quintets is to high field. The ^{11}B spectrum (b) is basically a triplet of triplets. Both this and (a) however contain second-order splittings. The figures around the formula give the various coupling constants. H_t are terminal and H_b are bridge hydrogen atoms respectively. (After Farrar, Johannensen and Coyle (1968) *J. Chem. Phys.*, **49**, 281, with permission.)

diborane containing the normal 19.6% of ^{10}B. The boron spectrum is basically a triplet of triplets arising from two isochronous boron atoms which are each coupled to two terminal protons and, by a smaller amount, to the two bridge protons. The proton spectrum consists basically of a 1:1:1:1 quartet to low field due to the terminal protons, which each have a major spin coupling to one boron atom, and a 1:2:3:4:3:2:1 septet of half the intensity to high field due to the bridge protons which are coupled equally to both boron atoms. The bridge protons also have a small spin coupling to all the terminal protons and each line of the septet is further split into a 1:4:6:4:1 quintet. Both the terminal proton quartet and the ^{11}B spectrum contain fine structure due to second-order spin coupling which arises because both the ^{11}B atoms and the terminal protons are not magnetically equivalent and the main peak separations are given by $^{1}J(B-H_t) + {}^{3}J(B-H_t)$. The spectrum can only be reconciled with the structure shown in the figure.

^{11}B NMR is also used extensively in the investigation of the higher polyhedral hydrides of boron and of the carboranes, compounds in which one or more of the boron atoms in a hydride have been replaced by carbon. Here we give one example of how the ^{11}B spectrum was used to determine the position in which two decaborane molecules may be joined to form the dimer. The decaborane molecule is a cluster of ten boron atoms placed approximately on ten of the twelve apices of an icosahedron. The structure is shown in Fig. 9.37. Each boron is bonded to a single hydrogen atom and the remaining four hydrogens form bridges as shown. The ^{11}B spectrum obtained at 115 MHz is shown with and without proton broad band irradiation. There are four types of boron in the molecule, each coupled to a single proton. The assignments to each position are shown on the spectra and the chemical shifts of course allow us to distinguish similar environments in related molecules. Two decaborane molecules can be joined together to form a dimer $B_{20}H_{26}$ connected by a boron–boron bond. Any of the boron atoms may be so involved and they need not be at the same position in the two halves of the dimer, so that eleven isomers are possible. These can be distinguished on the basis of their different ^{11}B spectra using the fact that the bonded borons will have singlet resonances in the absence of proton double irradiation and so can be identified by comparing spectra with and without irradiation. The spectra and crystal structure of the 2,2′ isomer are shown in Fig. 9.38. It is clear that only the 2-boron is unchanged on irradiation and that the 6,9-borons are now differentiated. The spectrum of another isomer is

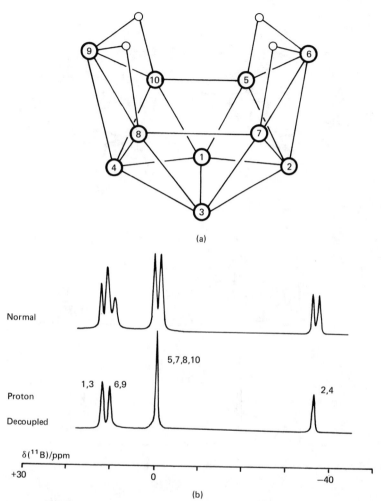

Figure 9.37 (a) The structure of decaborane. The large circles denote boron atoms, each of which carries a single hydrogen atom (not shown) and there are four hydrogen atoms which form boron–boron bridges, indicated by the small circles, to give the formula $B_{10}H_{14}$. There are four different types of boron site; 1 and 3, 2 and 4, 6 and 9, and the four positions 5, 7, 8, 10, so that the ^{11}B spectrum should contain four resonances in the intensity ratio 1:1:1:2 each split into a doublet by coupling to the terminal hydrogen atom. The bridge hydrogens have no observable effect on the spectrum.

(b) The 115 MHz ^{11}B spectra of decaborane with and without broad band double irradiation of the protons. The assignment of the resonances is given on the decoupled spectrum.

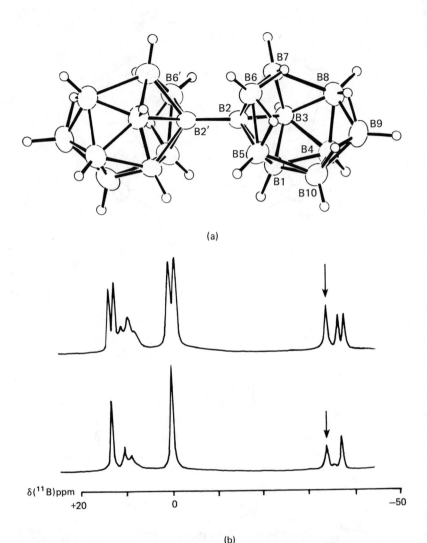

(a)

$\delta(^{11}B)$ppm

+20   0   −50

(b)

Figure 9.38 (a) One possible structure of the dimer of decarborane in which the boron–boron bond is formed between the two 2- positions.

(b) The ^{11}B spectra of the 2,2′ isomer. Only one resonance is unchanged upon proton double irradiation. Clearly, the chemical shifts are very little altered when the dimer forms so that we can conclude that the 2 position in each half of the dimer has lost its hydrogen and that this is where the boron–boron bond has formed. This conclusion was confirmed from the crystal structure. We note also that the neighbouring 6-boron is perturbed by the substitution at the 2- position.

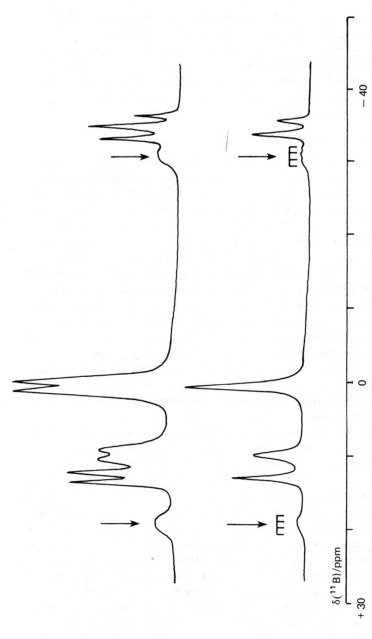

Figure 9.39 ^{11}B spectra of another $B_{20}H_{26}$ isomer. Two resonances remain unaffected by double irradiation and in this case show signs of partially collapsed ^{11}B—^{11}B coupling.

$\delta(^{11}B)/ppm$

shown in Fig. 9.39 and in this case two boron resonances remain unaffected by double irradiation and show partially collapsed boron–boron coupling. The three resonances to high field confirm that only one 2-boron is involved. The areas of the lines to low field show that there are still four 6,9 borons but only three 1,3 borons still coupled to a proton and the two halves of the dimer must in this case be coupled via the 1,2' atoms.

9.11.2   The aluminium-27 resonance

This is being used extensively to study the interactions occurring in ionic solutions since the rates of exchange around the triply charged cations are relatively slow and separate species can often be observed. Fig. 9.40 shows typical spectra obtained from an anhydrous methyl cyanide solution containing aluminium chloride and some aluminium perchlorate. Extensive ion pairing occurs and several distinct anions and cations are formed from the Al^{3+}. Resonances due to $AlCl_4^-$, $AlCl(MeCN)_5^{2+}$, $Al(MeCN)_6^{3+}$ (this at highest field), $Al(ClO_4)(MeCN)_5^{2+}$ and $Al(ClO_4)_2(MeCN)_4^+$ can be seen. A single Cl^- ligand causes a marked increase in the ^{27}Al relaxation rate, as would be expected from the decrease in symmetry around the aluminium. In contrast the perchlorate anion, which is a very effective ligand in this medium, has negligible effect on the line-width and presumably produces an electronic density at Al similar to that due to MeCN. The spectrum obtained from a solution containing only the perchlorate is also shown and indicates that complexes are formed containing three and four perchlorate anions.

The hydrolysis of $Al(H_2O)_6^{3+}$ has also been studied using the ^{27}Al resonance. The product of hydrolysis is often depicted as being $Al(H_2O)_5OH^{2+}$ though this is only ever a minor component and dimerizes to form $(H_2O)_4Al(\mu\text{-}OH)_2Al(H_2O)_2^{4+}$ with the aluminium ions bridged by two hydroxide ions. The dimer is formed in quantity if hydrolysis is forced by adding base (commonly as Na_2CO_3) and the two resonances are seen in Fig. 9.41. It is possible to remove a total of 2.5 protons per aluminium ion by adding further base and this causes further aggregation of dimer ions, probably around $Al(OH)_4^-$ ions formed as base is added, to form the cation $AlO_4Al_{12}(OH)_{24}(H_2O)_{12}^{7+}$ in which six dimer ions are arranged regularly around a central, tetrahedrally coordinated aluminium. Two resonances are observed, a sharp one due to the tetrahedral Al and a broad one due to the octahedral Al, whose octahedra are distorted by their need to wrap around the central Al. The spectra are used to follow the course of the hydrolysis reaction. It was found that the Al_{13} polymer was unstable and that prolonged hydrolysis or heating caused changes in the spectra, a typical one being shown at the bottom of the figure.

9.12 Main group V

Both nitrogen and phosphorus have been much studied. Nitrogen-14 has a quadrupole moment and gives rather broad lines in many of its compounds. Consequently much effort has been put into studies using the spin $\frac{1}{2}$ isotope nitrogen-15. In favourable cases it can be studied at natural abundance (0.635%) but ^{15}N enriched materials are commonly used. Phosphorus-31 on the other hand is a high receptivity spin $\frac{1}{2}$ nucleus and has been used by NMR spectroscopists right from the beginnings of the technique, and we will describe some results here.

9.12.1 The nitrogen-15 resonance

Two examples in which enriched ^{15}N has been used are shown in Figs. 9.42 and 9.43. In the first case the ^{15}N shift is sensitive to the isotopic composition of the molecule and the second gives confirmatory evidence for the structure of an ion containing only sulphur and nitrogen. The use of enriched material allows easy detection of a weak resonance in the first case and the detection of $^{15}N-^{15}N$ spin–spin coupling in the second.

9.12.2 The phosphorus-31 resonance

This has proved to be extremely useful in gaining information about metal-phosphine complexes. Fig. 9.44 shows a selectively decoupled ^{31}P spectrum of the iridium hydride

$$IrH_4R_2\overline{PCH_2}\overline{CHMeCHCH_2}\overline{CH_2PR_2}$$

where R = *t*-butyl. The phosphorus atoms and the carbon bonded to iridium are co-planar, with the former *trans*. Because the two rings thus formed are different, the four hydride hydrogen atoms should be non-equivalent. However, provided the ^{31}P spectrum is simplified by selectively irradiating the protons bonded to carbon atoms, each component of its AB quartet is found to consist of a 1:4:6:4:1 quintet showing that either phosphorus atom is coupled equally to the four

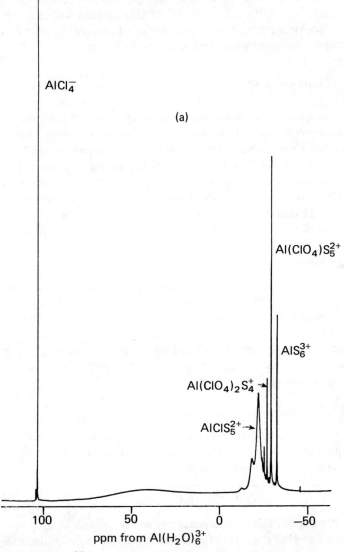

Figure 9.40 ^{27}Al spectra at 104.2 MHz of aluminium salts dissolved in methyl cyanide. (a) A mixture of $AlCl_3$ and $Al(ClO_4)_3$. Eight species of ion are present, the formulae of the five of greatest concentration being marked by their respective resonances. S signifies the solvent MeCN. Small amounts of ions containing three perchlorate ligands or two or three chloride ligands are also present. The broad line in the centre of the spectrum is due to an Al containing solid in the spectrometer probe.

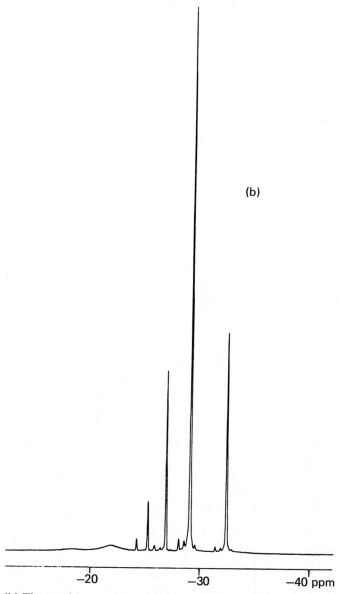

(b) The perchlorate salt, contaminated with a small amount of chloride to give the broad resonance, but showing that 1,2,3 or four solvent ligands can be replaced by ClO_4^-. The assignment is based on the fact that the chemical shifts are characteristic of octahedral Al and that proton NMR gives a solvation number between 5 and 6. The small sharp peaks are spinning side bands.

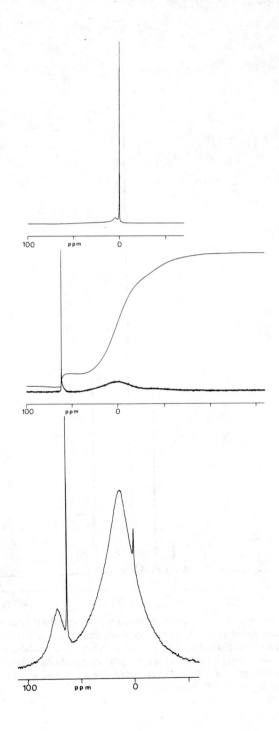

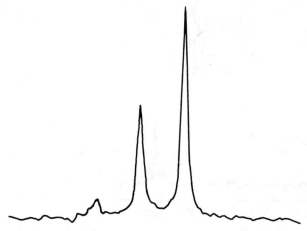

Figure 9.42 The ^{15}N NMR spectrum of the nitrite ion NO_2^- in water. The ion was enriched to 95% in ^{15}N and 77% in ^{18}O. The three resonances arise from ions of isotopic composition $^{15}N^{16}O_2$, $^{15}N^{16,18}O$ and $^{15}N^{18}O_2$ in the concentration ratios 6:33:61. Replacement of ^{16}O by ^{18}O causes an upfield shift of 0.138 ppm. (Reproduced with permission from Van Etten and Risley (1981) *J. Amer. Chem. Soc.*, **103**, 5633.)

hydride protons. This feature persists to at least $-100°$C and shows that the hydride hydrogen atoms are rapidly interchanging their positions to give equal, average coupling to the ^{31}P.

If the iridium complex *mer*-Ir(PMe$_3$)$_3$Cl$_3$ is treated with base then a chloride ion and a proton are extracted, the latter of course coming from a methyl group which then forms a bond to the vacant coordination site on the metal to give a three membered IrPC ring. The ^{31}P$\{^1$H$\}$

Figure 9.41 ^{27}Al spectra at 104.2 MHz of hydrolysed aqueous aluminium chloride solutions. In the upper spectrum, sufficient Na$_2$CO$_3$ has been added to react with one hydrogen ion per aluminium ion and the solution contains Al(H$_2$O)$_6^{3+}$ (sharp line at 0 ppm) and the dihydroxy bridged dimer, whose line is broader because the bridging distorts the octahedra. If Na$_2$CO$_3$ is added to react with 2.5 H$^+$ per Al^{3+} then a polymer is formed containing 13 aluminium ions in different environments in the ratio 1:12. One Al is tetrahedrally coordinated and gives a narrow line and the remainder reside in distorted octahedra and give a broad line (central spectrum). The lower spectrum shows how the decomposition of this polymeric ion leads to marked changes in the spectra. (Reproduced with permisson from Akitt and Mann (1981) *J. Mag. Res.*, **44**, 584.)

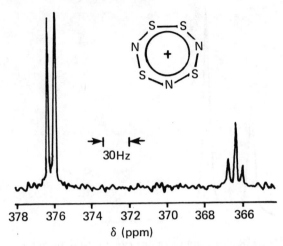

Figure 9.43   The ^{15}N NMR spectrum of 99% ^{15}N enriched S_4N_3Cl (0.2 M in 70% HNO_3) proving the presence of two chemically different types of nitrogen in a 2:1 atomic ratio. (Reproduced with permission from Chivers *et al.* (1981) *Inorg. Chem.*, **20**, 914.)

spectrum of this product is shown in Fig. 9.45 and is an ABC pattern with one large *trans* coupling of 354 Hz and two *cis* couplings of nominally 35 and 8 Hz. The phosphorus in the ring has a markedly different shift to the other two. If the phosphines were all *cis* (the *fac* complex), no large P–P coupling would be observed.

Our next example illustrates both the sort of spectra obtainable from these complexes and how in some cases their formation may be followed in detail. An oxidative addition was carried out on the platinum complex $PtMe_2(Me_2PC_6H_3(OMe)_2)_2$ using benzyl bromide, with the objective of forming the octahedral complex $PtMe_2(Me_2PC_6-H_3(OMe)_2)_2(PhCH_2)Br$, where Ph = a phenyl group. The proton decoupled ^{31}P spectrum of the starting material is shown in Fig. 9.46 and is the typical 1:4:1 triplet (see Fig. 9.23). The initial product has a similar spectrum though with different shift and coupling constant but, even after $1\frac{1}{2}$ hours reaction there is already a significant amount of another product present. After three days this becomes a predominant spectral feature and is seen to consist of 1:4:1 set of AB sub spectra. The initial product has isomerized to give non-equivalent phosphines which have a small *cis* P–P coupling. The full structure can then be deduced from the methyl resonance pattern in the ^1H spectrum

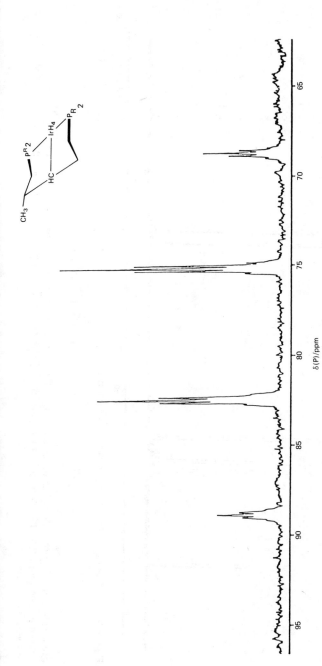

$\delta(P)/ppm$

Figure 9.44   The ^{31}P spectrum at 40.5 MHz of the complex iridium hydride $IrH_4\{Bu_2^t PCH_2 CHMeCHCH_2 CH_2 PBu_2^t\}$ with those protons which are bonded directly to carbon selectively decoupled so that only the protons on the iridium can spin couple to the phosphorus. The two phosphorus atoms of the phosphine ligand are non equivalent because of the methyl group substituent in one half of the ligand and so can show a large *trans* coupling to give an AB quartet. Each line of this quartet is a quintet and so is coupled equally to four spin $\frac{1}{2}$ nuclei; namely the four protons. The reference in this and all the following ^{31}P spectra is external 85% *ortho*-phosphoric acid.

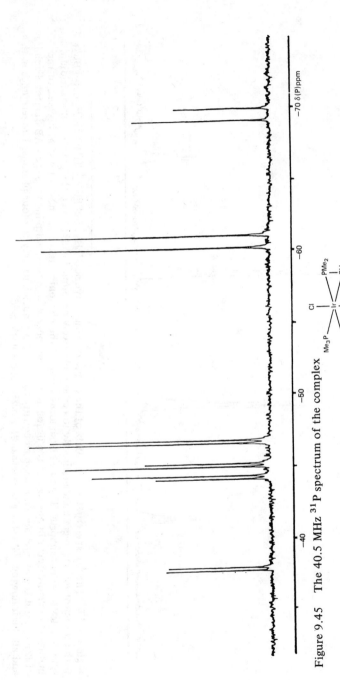

Figure 9.45 The 40.5 MHz ^{31}P spectrum of the complex

obtained with full proton broad band decoupling. All splittings in the three resonances are due to ^{31}P—^{31}P spin–spin coupling. The multiplet at −45 ppm is the C part of the ABC spectrum and so has an unusual intensity pattern since it lies within the AB part.

which contains one large and one small coupling; hence one *cis* and one *trans* methyl group.

Phosphorus chemistry is also very important in biological studies. One key compound is adenosine tri-phosphate (ATP) which is involved in the production of bio-energy but which needs the intervention of magnesium ions. Fig. 9.47 shows the spectra of a pure ATP solution and a series with added Mg^{2+}. Three resonances are observed corresponding to the three phosphorus atoms in the phosphate chain and these are split by two-bond phosphorus–phosphorus coupling. The resulting multiplet pattern allows the resonances to be assigned to individual atoms. The resonance at highest field is a triplet and so must be the central, β phosphorus. The doublet to low field shows extra, though poorly resolved coupling to two protons and so must be the α phosphorus. The ^1H–^{31}P coupling is removed by proton double irradiation. The lowest field doublet is then the end γ phosphorus atom. The effect of the Mg^{2+} was studied by obtaining spectra with the spectrometer locked to D_2O in the solvent which then became a secondary standard, and was calibrated by obtaining a spectrum of an orthophosphoric acid solution. The effect of the added metal ion is quite curious and influences both the chemical shifts and the coupling between the phosphorus atoms. Only one set of resonances is observed so that any complexed ATP must be in rapid exchange with the free form. All resonances move downfield with small additions of Mg^{2+}, the effect being least for the α atoms, and reach a limiting shift when one Mg^{2+} has been added per ATP molecule. The coupling constant also falls from 19.5 Hz to 15 Hz indicating that the conformation of the chain is changed by the formation of the complex. Further addition of magnesium however reverses these chemical shift changes but leaves the coupling constant reduced. The chain conformation must thus remain constrained by complexation and more magnesium must be thus remain constrained by complexation and more magnesium must be complexed to form a 2:1 complex. The upfield shift caused by the second magnesium ion can be explained by its complexing on the other side of the phosphate chain, where there are several unused oxygen donor groups, which may well reduce the p electron imbalance around the phosphorus atoms and so reduce the paramagnetic contribution to the shift.

9.13   Main group VI

9.13.1   Oxygen-17 spectroscopy

Like nitrogen-15, oxygen-17 is naturally of low abundance and so is

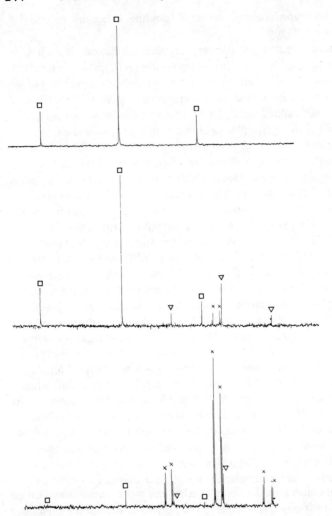

Figure 9.46   Three 40.5 MHz ^{31}P spectra obtained with proton broad band irradiation which show the progress of an oxidative addition to a platinum complex.

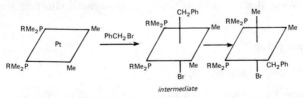

where R = $C_6H_3(OMe_2)_2$ and Ph = phenyl.

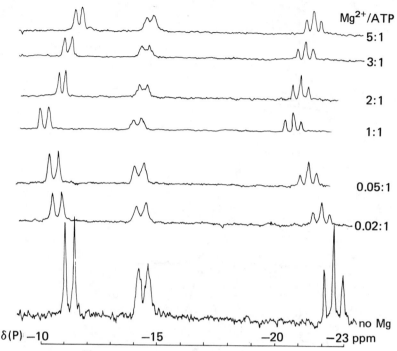

Figure 9.47 ^{31}P FT spectra of solutions of ATP dissolved in H_2O/D_2O alone and with added $MgCl_2$ at the mole ratios shown beside each spectrum. The shifts are relative to external H_3PO_4. Starting from highest field, the resonances are assigned to the β (triplet), α (showing a small coupling to the methylene protons) and γ phosphorus atoms. The two ^{31}P–^{31}P coupling constants are equal in all these solutions. The structural formula is shown below. (Akitt and Birch, unpublished results.)

The upper trace is from the initial material and is marked by squares in the following spectra. The centre trace, taken 1½ hours after the reactants had been mixed, contains a similar triplet pattern of a product (triangles) and a minor component, marked X. After three days reaction the predominant spectrum is that marked X which shows extra coupling to give a triplet of AB patterns which indicate that the phosphines are no longer equivalent. This product is formed via an intermediate as depicted in the reaction scheme above.

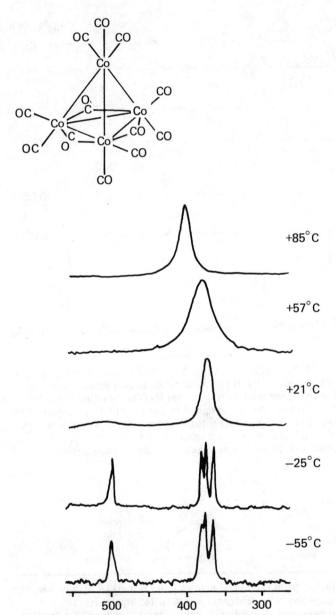

Figure 9.48   The oxygen-17 spectrum of $(CO)_{12}Co_4$. The carbonyl groups exchange positions but this can be slowed down sufficiently by cooling to enable the four types of carbonyl group to be seen. The reference is water. (Reproduced with permission from Aime *et al*. (1981) *J. Amer. Chem. Soc.*, **103**, 5920.)

commonly used in an enriched form. It is a quadrupolar nucleus but gives reasonably narrow lines in many environments, while its relaxation times are quite short so that data can be collected at a high rate and compensate for a normally small enrichment level, made necessary by the high cost of the enriched isotope. The example in Fig. 9.48 shows some ^{17}O spectra obtained over a range of temperatures from a solution of the cobalt complex $(CO)_{12}Co_4$. The carbonyl groups interchange position rapidly on the NMR time scale at high temperatures but the rate of exchange becomes sufficiently slow at $-25°$ for the resonances of the four types of carbonyl to be resolved, with the bridging groups well to low field. The carbon spectrum will of course give the same information as the oxygen spectrum but interestingly in this case the latter gives a much wider chemical shift dispersion for what are identical ligands in rather similar environments.

The cobalt-59 spectrum of this compound has also been obtained and contains two resonances in the expected 3:1 intensity ratio. This nucleus also relaxes by the quadrupolar mechanism so that the irregular stereochemistry around the cobalt atoms means that the lines are very broad at about 7500 Hz.

9.14   Main group VII

9.14.1   Fluorine-19 NMR

The fluorine-19 nucleus is also an important one since it is 100% abundant and gives a signal intensity second only to that of the proton. It is a spin $\frac{1}{2}$ nucleus and its spectroscopy is very similar to that of the proton except that the chemical shifts between fluorine atoms in different environments in a molecule are often very large. If spin coupling exists then first-order patterns are obtained. A large number of compounds has been studied but here we can give only a very superficial glance at a major area of NMR spectroscopy.

The first example concerns the tetrafluoroborate anion BF_4^-. The fluorine atoms are arranged tetrahedrally around the boron so that the electric field gradient at the boron nucleus is small and electric quadrupole relaxation is slight. Thus the boron spin coupling to the fluorine atoms can be observed in the fluorine spectrum. This consists of a well-resolved quartet due to the 80.6% of $^{11}BF_4^-$ ions (boron-11, $I = \frac{3}{2}$) and a septet due to the 19.4% of $^{10}BF_4^-$ (boron-10, $I = 3$) (Fig. 9.49). The spectrum is particularly interesting in that it clearly demonstrates that the fluorine atoms attached to the boron isotope ^{11}B are chemically shifted from those attached to ^{10}B. This is called an isotope shift and arises because the vibrational states of the two ions

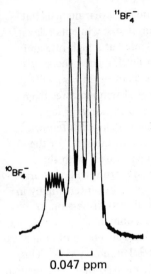

0.047 ppm

Figure 9.49   Fluorine-19 spectrum of the BF_4^- ion in an aqueous solution of ammonium tetrafluoroborate. The septet at low field arises from fluorine bonded to the isotope ^{10}B ($I = 3$) and the quartet at high field from fluorine bonded to ^{11}B ($I = \frac{3}{2}$). The different isotopic masses cause a fluorine chemical shift of 0.047 ppm. The coupling constants are ^1J ($^{11}B-^{19}F$) = 1.2 Hz; ^1J ($^{10}B-^{19}F$) = 0.4 Hz.

differ slightly so that the electron distributions within the bonds are also different (see Fig. 9.42 for a more recent example).

The coupling constants to the two isotopes should be in the ratio of the magnetogyric ratios which is $\gamma(^{10}B)/\gamma(^{11}B) = 0.335$. The corresponding coupling constants are found to be in the ratio 0.33.

The ion is unusual in that the coupling constant varies over a considerable range depending on its environment. In aqueous NH_4BF_4, $^1J(^{11}B-^{19}F)$ is 1.2 Hz whereas in $NaBF_4$ solution it may attain values of up to 5.0 Hz, depending upon the concentration. In non-aqueous solvents the coupling constant may change sign. This behaviour is thought to arise because of the presence of two large electronic contributions to the coupling constant which are opposite in sign and therefore nearly cancel. Changes in environment produce small but different changes in each contribution which are large in relation to the net coupling constant and so become particularly obvious.

The second example is of the spectrum of methylaminotetrafluoro-phosphorane, CH_3NHPF_4 which is prepared by reaction between $CH_3NHSi(CH_3)$ and PF_5. A singlet is observed at 70° suggesting that all the fluorine atoms exist in the same environment. No resonance

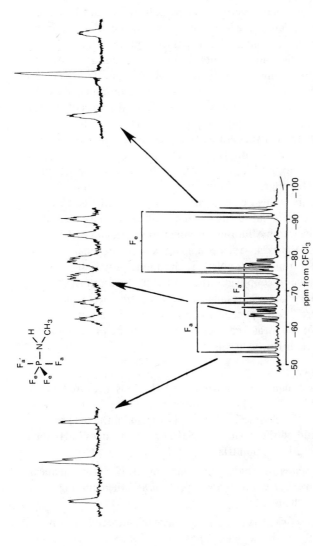

Figure 9.50 The lower trace shows the full ^{19}F spectrum of $(CH_3)NHPF_4$ at $-80°$. The resonances of three types of fluorine atom in 1:1:2 ratio are split into doublets by coupling to phosphorus. One member of each doublet is shown in expanded form in the upper traces. The probable stereochemistry is shown in the formula. The data extracted from the spectrum are: chemical shifts, $Fa = -60$, $Fa' = -70$ and $Fe = -83$ ppm from $CFCl_3$; coupling constants, $^1J(PFa) = 755$, $^1J(PFa') = 770$, $^1J(PFe) = 920$, $^2J(FaFe) = 68$, $^2J(Fa'Fe) = 69$, $^2J(FaFa') = 2.8$, $^3J(Fa'NH) = 27.6$, $^4J(Fa'CH) = 2.8$ and $^4J(FeCH) = 2.1$ Hz. Coupling to ^{31}P is also observed in the proton spectrum and $^2J(PNH) = 21$ and $^3J(PCH) = 15.2$ Hz. (Reproduced with permission from Harman and Sharp (1971) *Inorg. Chem.*, **10**, 1538.)

is detectable at $30°$ suggesting that an exchange process is causing averaging of differing fluorine environments and indeed, further cooling to $-80°$ causes a complex spectrum to emerge as shown in Fig. 9.50. This contains three identical pairs of multiplets, each pair arising from phosphorus–fluorine coupling. This means that there are three distinguishable fluorine environments. These compounds are known to adopt a trigonal bipyramid stereochemistry which means that wherever the amine is placed, there should be two fluorine environments, axial or equatorial. We see usually equal numbers of the two sorts of fluorine so that the ligands take an equatorial position as shown in the figure. The singlet at $70°$ then arises because the axial and equatorial fluorine atoms can interchange position. However, in this case a second process must also intervene to produce the splitting into three resonances in the ratio $1:1:2$. This appears to be a freezing of the rotation of the amine ligand and its taking up an orientation such that the two axial fluorine atoms are non-equivalent. All three resonances have a basic triplet structure caused by fluorine–fluorine coupling, and restricted to triplets because the axial–axial coupling is small. One axial triplet is further split into a triplet of doublets by the amino proton and fine structure is seen due to coupling to the methyl protons and the other axial fluorine. The equatorial resonances also contain unresolved coupling and there is some general second-order perturbation of the intensities, so that the measured coupling constants are probably not exactly equal to their true values.

Further exercises

1   The proton resonance of chloroform, $CHCl_3$, was measured as 730 Hz downfield of TMS. The spectrometer operating frequency was 100 MHz. What is the chemical shift of chloroform on the δ and τ scales? What would be the separation of the two resonances in Hz for a spectrometer operating at 60 MHz?

2   Fig. 3.5 illustrates an ethyl group spectrum. Measure the chemical shifts (δ) of the methyl and methylene protons and the coupling constant between them.

3   A sketch of the 40 MHz proton resonance of tetraethyl lead is shown in Fig. 9.51, with the relative positions of each line marked in Hz (assuming first-order line positions). Lead contains the following isotopes:

^{206}Pb natural abundance 24% $I = 0$
^{207}Pb natural abundance 22% $I = \frac{1}{2}$
^{208}Pb natural abundance 54% $I = 0$

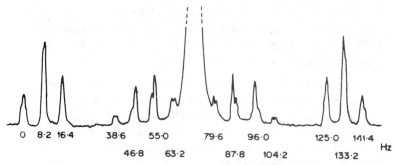

Figure 9.51   40 MHz proton spectrum of tetraethyl lead. (After Narasimhan and Rogers (1961) *J. Chem. Phys.*, 34, 1049, with permission.)

Explain the various features of the spectrum and calculate the coupling constants between lead and the methyl and methylene protons and also the interproton coupling constant. What is the chemical shift between the methyl and methylene protons?

The satellite line intensities are perturbed from the theoretical so that the spectrum is slightly second order. This is also evident in the tendency for extra splittings to appear in the quartet–triplet patterns. The effect is nevertheless only slight and can be shown to conform to the expected pattern for a separation equal to that between a methyl triplet one one side of the central resonance and a methylene quartet on the opposite side. What does this tell us about the relative signs of $^2J(^{207}\text{Pb}–^1\text{H})$ and $^3J(^{207}\text{Pb}–^1\text{H})$? Suggest why $^3J > {}^2J$.

4   Fig. 3.14c shows the spectrum of ascaridole. The spectrum features a closely coupled AB quartet at about δ = 6.45 ppm. The line positions, starting at the lowest field, are 395.5, 386.9, 385.5, and 376.9 Hz from TMS. Calculate $^3J(\text{H}_c–\text{H}_d)$ and the chemical shift between H_c and H_d in Hz.

5   Fig. 7.5 shows the proton spectrum of pentadeutero dimethyl-sulphoxide, CD_3SOCD_2H. The two deuterons split the proton resonance into a quintet. What should the relative intensities of the five lines be? What is $^2J(\text{H–H})$ in the methyl group, given $^2J(\text{H–D})$ = 1.85 Hz.

6   Construct a stick diagram for the fluorine and borane proton resonances of the complex adduct $HF_2P \cdot BH_3$ given that $^1J(^{11}\text{B–H})$ = 103 Hz. $^3J(\text{F–H})$ = 26 Hz, $^2J(\text{P–H})$ = 17.5 Hz, $^3J(\text{H–H})$ = 4.0 Hz, $^1J(\text{P–F})$ = 1151 Hz and $^2J(\text{H–F})$ = 54.5 Hz.

7   The proton resonances of TMS and cyclohexane are separated by
1.43 ppm the cyclohexane being to low field. If the TMS resonates at
60 000 000 Hz in a particular field locked spectrometer, at what
frequency will the cyclohexane resonate?

8   The fluorine resonance of the hexafluoroniobate ion $^{93}NbF_6^-$
observed as a viscous solution in dimethylformamide is a well-resolved
multiplet at 60°C. The spin of ^{93}Nb is 9/2. How many lines should be
observed in the multiplet? If the sample is cooled to 0°C or heated to
125°C the multiplicity is lost and a broad unresolved resonance is
obtained. Explain these observations.

9   Fig. 9.52 shows the fluorine-19 resonance of the CF_2H group of
1, 1, 1, 2, 2, 3, 3-heptafluoropropane, $CF_3CF_2CF_2H$. The two
fluorines are equivalent and are coupled to all the other magnetically
active nuclei in the sample. Pick out the various multiplet patterns and
measure the coupling constants $^2J(F-H)$, $^3J(F-F)$, and $^4J(F-F)$.

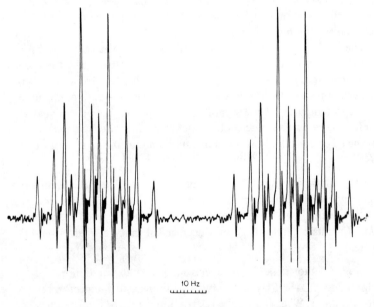

10 Hz

Figure 9.52 ^{19}F resonance of the CF_2H group of $CF_3CF_2CF_2H$.

10   The proton spectrum of a sample of neat methanol, CH_3OH
consists at 20°C of two singlets with the hydroxyl resonance 1.6 ppm
low field of the methyl resonance. If the temperature is progressively
reduced the singlets broaden; structure appears and at −60° C the

hydroxyl resonance is a 1:3:3:1 quartet and the methyl resonance is a doublet. In addition the hydroxyl resonance moves downfield and is now 2.3 ppm from the methyl doublet. Explain these observations.

11   Fig. 3.7e shows the methyl proton spectrum of $[Me_2NBCl_2]_2$ and ascribes it to spin spin coupling to two ^{11}B nuclei. The presence of 19.6% of ^{10}B in the molecules is said to lead to line broadening. About 39% of the molecules will contain one ^{10}B atom and one ^{11}B atom. Construct a stick diagram for the methyl resonances of these molecules and show how this reduces the resolution of the all ^{11}B septet. The spin of ^{11}B is $\frac{3}{2}$ and of ^{10}B is 3.

12   Explain why in Figs 3.14a and b the two halves of the AB quartets have different intensities.

13   Use the figures in the table given on p. 226 for the rates of exchange of Na^+ between free ionic state and bound to the cryptand to obtain the activation energy of the process.

14   Fig. 9.53 shows the ^1H spectrum obtained at 60 MHz of the

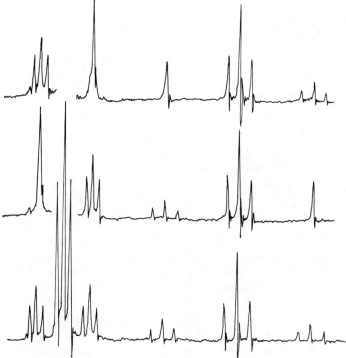

Figure 9.53   (Example supplied by J. D. Kennedy.)

methyl resonances of the complex $(Me_2C_6H_5P)_2PtMeCl$ in which the
two phosphine ligands are *trans*. The spectrum is closely similar to
that of the bromo complex shown in Fig. 9.25. The lower trace is the
single resonance spectrum and the upper two were obtained while
irradiating in the region of the ^{31}P frequency at 24.285 210 MHz
(upper trace) or 24.288 100 MHz (lower trace), and in each case
selective decoupling occurs. Explain the different origins of the various
triplet patterns in the single resonance spectrum. What do the
decoupled patterns tell us about the coupling between the platinum
and the methyl protons? Platinum contains 33.7% of the magnetically
active nucleus ^{195}Pt with $I = \frac{1}{2}$, the remaining isotopes having $I = 0$;
phosphorus is 100% ^{31}P with $I = \frac{1}{2}$ and the proton also has $I = \frac{1}{2}$. All
three isotopes have positive magnetogyric ratios.

15   An FT spectrometer is set up so that the carbon-13 spectrum of
a given sample has upright peaks for spectra obtained with a 90° pulse.
Will the peaks be upright or inverted for (a) a 30° pulse (b) a 150°
pulse (c) a 180° pulse (d) a 210° pulse (e) a 330° pulse? What are the
relative absolute intensities?

16   A sample gives a free induction decay in an FT spectrometer
operating at 60 MHz which contains an obvious beat pattern with the
beat maxima separated by 0.2 s. A beat pattern with the same
separation between maxima was also evident when the sample was
placed in a 100 MHz spectrometer. What does this tell us about the
resonances giving rise to the beat pattern?

17   Fig. 7.17 illustrates how a slow exchange process may be
measured. Given that T_1 for the 2,6 carbon atoms is 0.64 s, calculate
the average lifetime of one conformation at 226 K. Use a ruler to obtain
the relative equilibrium magnetizations.

18   It is desired to obtain the spectra of a series of samples in a
certain Fourier transform spectrometer with a magnetic field such that
the resonance of highest frequency is likely to be at 100.010 00 MHz
and that of lowest frequency at 100.000 00 MHz. To what frequency
should the spectrometer be set to ensure that all resonances appear to
'high field' of the spectrometer frequency? What dwell time should be
used to ensure that all signals are shown in their correct frequency
relationship and are not folded? If the free induction decay were taken
in 16 K of memory, what then is the minimum line separation which
can be observed, i.e. what is the resolution of the system? If each
sample required 1000 decays to be added before a satisfactory signal to
noise ratio were obtained, how long would it take to run each sample?

Answers

1   δ = 7.3 ppm τ = 2.7   438 Hz

2   Chemical shifts are 1.48 and 3.56 ppm
    $^3J(H–H)$ = 7 Hz

3   $^3J(H–H)$ = 8.2 Hz $^3J(Pb–H)$ = 125.0 Hz $^2J(Pb–H)$ = 41.0 Hz
    methyl–methylene shift = 0.0175 ppm
    methylene protons to high field

4   J = 8.6 Hz, shift = 5.1 Hz

5   1:2:3:2:1, 12.05 Hz.

6   The proton resonance contains 48 lines and the fluorine
    resonance, where some lines overlap, contains only 12 lines. The
    spectra are illustrated in the *Journal of the Americal Chemical
    Society*, **89**, pp. 1622–1623.

7   The resonances are separated by 85.8 Hz at 60 MHz. The
    cyclohexane protons are less screened, experience the larger
    applied magnetic field and so always precess at a higher
    frequency than do the protons in TMS.

8   The multiplicity is ten. The loss of resolution at one extreme is
    due to quadrupole relaxation and at the other extreme to
    exchange of fluoride ion, involving Nb–F bond breaking.

9   The pattern is a doublet of quartets of triplets with coupling
    constants of 53 Hz, 7.3 Hz, and 4.7 Hz. No lines overlap.

10 The hydroxyl proton is exchanging. Its chemical shift is
    determined by the degree of hydrogen bonding it experiences.

11 A 1:1:1:2:2:3:2:2:3:2:2:2:1:1:1 multiplet is obtained. None
    of the lines coincide with those of the all ^{11}B multiplet.

12 Because in (a) the H(c) resonance is broadened slightly by
    coupling to the methyl group and in (b) H(c) is broadened
    slightly by coupling to the ring nitrogen.

13 The activation energy is 51 kJ mol^{-1}.

14 The spectrum contains two groups of multiplets, one to high
    field due to the methyl directly bonded to platinum and one to
    low field due to the phosphine methyl groups. Each is made up
    of a 1:4:1 triplet pattern with a central group arising from the

complexes with magnetically inactive platinum and satellites due to those containing ^{195}Pt. Each of these lines is split into a triplet by coupling to two ^{31}P nuclei, though for the phosphine methyl groups this involves virtual coupling, and so a *trans* arrangement of phosphines. The phosphorus spectrum is of course split into a 1:4:1 set of multiplets by the platinum and if one of the ^{195}Pt satellites is weakly irradiated at the phosphorus frequency, then any perturbation of coupled resonances is limited to those attached to the ^{195}Pt with the same spin orientation. In other words the platinum coupling splits the population of our sample into three distinguishable parts. Irradiating the low frequency satellite in the ^{31}P spectrum affects the low frequency PMe triplet and the high frequency PtMe triplet. This means that the ^{195}Pt spin state which gives a low frequency ^{31}P satellite gives high frequency PtMe and low frequency PMe satellites. Thus the signs of ^1J(PtP) and ^3J(PtPCH) are the same and opposite to that of ^2J(PtCH).

15 All outputs will have the same absolute intensity except for (c) which will be zero. (a) and (b) will be upright and (d) and (e) will be inverted.

16 The spectrum must contain a strong component which is a multiplet with line separations of 5 Hz. This separation is not field dependant and so must be due to spin–spin coupling. It is also likely that the nucleus causing the splitting is not the same species as the one observed.

17 $\tau = 0.39$ s or thereabouts.

18 Spectrometer frequency = 100.010 00 MHz. A spectral width of at least 10 000 Hz required which means a dwell time of 50 μs. After Fourier transformation the absorption part of the transformation is contained in half the memory, i.e. 8K or 8192 memory locations. The resolution is then 10 000/8192 Hz/ location or 1.22 Hz. The time taken to collect one decay is 16 384 x 50 μs. 1000 accumulations therefore takes 819.2 s or about $13\frac{2}{3}$ minutes.

Bibliography

Because of the importance and utility of NMR spectroscopy a very considerable number of books, articles and reviews have been published covering various aspects of the subject within the last thirty years. A recent review of the literature lists seventy titles, several of which are of series appearing annually. The following list represents only a fraction of the total but is sufficient to give an entry into the field.

Four comprehensive works are available for general reference.

Pople, J. A., Schneider, W. G. and Bernstein, H. J. (1959), *High Resolution Nuclear Magnetic Resonance*, McGraw-Hill, New York.
Emsley, J. W., Feeney, J. and Sutcliffe, L. H. (1965), *High Resolution Nuclear Magnetic Resonance Spectroscopy* in two volumes; Pergamon Press, Oxford.
Jackman, C. M. and Sternhell, S. (1969), *Applications of Nuclear Magnetic Resonance Spectroscopy in Organic Chemistry* 2nd Edn. In the International Series of Monographs in Organic Chemistry Volume 5, Pergamon Press, Oxford.
Abragam, A. (1961), *The Principles of Nuclear Magnetism*, Oxford.

Several books have been published which are introductory texts and some of which contain a variety of problems including the interpretation of spectral traces. Some are listed below and the student may find these or other similar in the library.

Abraham, R. J. and Loftus, P. (1978), *Proton and Carbon-13 NMR Spectroscopy—an integrated approach*, Heyden and Son Ltd, London.

Ault, A. and Ault, M. R. (1980), *A Handy and Systematic Catalog of NMR Spectra-Instruction through Examples*, University Science Books, California.

Gunther, H. (1973, translated 1980), *NMR Spectroscopy—an introduction*, John Wiley & Son, New York.

Levy, G. C., Lichter, R. C. and Nelson, G. L. (1980, second edition), *Carbon-13 NMR Spectroscopy*, John Wiley & Son, New York.

Lynden-Bell, R. M. and Harris, R. K. (1969), *Nuclear Magnetic Resonance Spectroscopy*, Nelson, London.

The techniques of NMR, including the Fourier transform methods are described in the following two books:

Martin, M. L., Delpuech, J.-J. and Martin, G. J. (1980), *Practical NMR Spectroscopy*, Heyden & Son Ltd, London.

Mullen, K. and Pregosin, P. S. (1976), *FT NMR Techniques—a practical approach*, Academic Press, London and New York.

The student may also care to read the following few original short papers which summarize the early and unexpected results which heralded the development of NMR as a subject useful to chemists.

Dickinson, W. C. (1950), *Phys. Revs.*, **77**, 736, Observed chemical shifts in fluorine compounds and noted the effect of exchange.

Proctor, W. G. and Yu, F. C. (1950), *Phys. Revs.*, **77**, 717, ^{14}N chemical shift between NH_4^+ and NO_3^-.

Arnold, J. T., Dharmatti, S. S., and Packard, M. E. (1951), *J. Chem. Phys.*, **19**, 507, First observation of chemical shifts in a single chemical compound.

Gutowsky, H. S., and McCall, D. W. (1951), *Phys. Revs.*, **82**, 748, An early observation of spin—spin coupling.

Gutowsky, H. S., McCall, D. W. and Slichter, C. P. (1951), *Phys. Revs.*, **84**, 589, A theory of spin—spin coupling.

It should be remembered in reading the last two papers that the Hz separation of the ^{31}P doublet and ^{19}F doublet are the same. The gauss separation can be calculated from $\Delta B_0 = (J/v_0)B_0$ and is greater for ^{31}P since v_0 is smaller for the fixed field used.

Index